FUTURISTIC HEALTH TODAY

SHERRY DELL

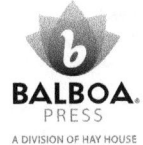

BALBOA.
PRESS

A DIVISION OF HAY HOUSE

Balboa Press books may be ordered through booksellers or by contacting:

Balboa Press
A Division of Hay House
1663 Liberty Drive
Bloomington, IN 47403
www.balboapress.com
1 (877) 407-4847

Print information available on the last page.

ISBN: 978-1-9822-2730-2 (sc)
ISBN: 978-1-9822-2729-6 (hc)
ISBN: 978-1-9822-2728-9 (e)

Library of Congress Control Number: 2019906860

Balboa Press rev. date: 05/15/2019

CONTENTS

DEDICATION

Edith Freeman Harris

December 12, 1920–April 24, 2018

For loving support as a mother and confidante who worked diligently the year my office opened in 2000. Mama, you helped me pray my way out of some serious illnesses. You stood behind me when I defied all odds of infertility and delivered, by natural birth, an eight-pound, two-ounce infant at the age of forty-four. You cared for him when my career was on fire, and I had to juggle my time at the clinic and home with a newborn. You introduced me to healing modalities and helped me secure my first job at Real-Life health food store. You listened to my logic as I unveiled mysteries of healing with the use of organic foods and vitamin supplements. You said, "Count me in, and give me the remedy." Because you believed in holistic medicine, you lived ninety-seven years young and passed away peacefully and cognizant until your last breath. May your music and laughter echo the gates of heaven.

PREFACE

When health is absent, wisdom cannot reveal itself, art cannot express itself, strength cannot be exerted ... And reason is powerless.

— Herophilus to Alexander the Great

My Childhood Gift

When I was four years old, one of the first memories I recall as a healer came when I was sitting in the third pew of Grace Baptist Church, where my parents, three siblings, and I attended church service in the late sixties. As I sat in my Sunday best, a dress Mama had just sewn for me, I would plead with myself not to look back at Mrs. Thompson. We had been scolded for staring at others, especially when they looked different, and Mrs. Thompson revealed an anomaly that was hard for a curious young girl like me to ignore. I remember thinking something had eaten that poor old woman's nose. My mother explained to me that Mrs. Thompson had been battling cancer, leaving her with only a semblance of a nose where two hollow holes bore into her sweet, reverent face. The inexplicable pain that took place when I peeked at her was why I so dreaded looking back at ol' Mrs. T. One glance would cause tremendous pain in my thighs. I would grab the bottom of my dress, but the pain would not relent. As I pressed on my thighs with my little hands clad in white gloves, I prayed to God for the pain to end.

As a very young child in that Baptist church filled with songs of praise, I was taught to pray for the sick and believed it was my duty. On quiet, sunny days in Texas, I packed a sack lunch and grape soda, hiked up the street, climbed the wooden stairs in the back of that same old Baptist church, and began my communion with God. I filled to the brim my emotional glass of optimism and seemed to have the clarity of specific healing taking place because of my asking. I thanked God always for answering my prayers and believed they were answered, period. I never lost the confidence in the sincere prayers I offered, and I believed with all my little-girl heart that people were healing daily. I knew then and I know now, spoken words of healing are powered by belief, enthusiasm, and songs of intention.

Meditation

Time passed by quickly as I began to meditate for a deeper connection to God. I progressively became aware of my medical intuitiveness. My own sickness of migraines, yeast infections, high blood pressure, thyroid tumors, hypoglycemia, and infertility drew me closer to fulfilling my future as a naturopathic healer. Eventually I learned to thank God for my illnesses because I viewed them as a gift and a challenge I could overcome. I prayed intensely over the sickness of migraines until God blessed me with the formula to heal them. I believe that 80 percent of migraines are caused by a congested liver. This congestion consists of an overload of food allergies, estrogen, processed foods, and chemicals from drugs.

Divine Guidance

Society was rapidly embracing health food and vitamins during the seventies and eighties. I'm sure I was called a health-food nut more than once. I now see how my path to healing was steered by the hands of God. I managed to obtain quite an extensive education for myself to serve and guide the sick folks sent my way. My vocation began with a license in massage therapy, foot reflexology, and a certification in designed clinical nutrition at Parker Chiropractic College in Irving, Texas. I was becoming a healer. My motto was: "To whom may I serve." I began a practice of saying this devotional phrase every day as I drove to work. I had read this passage in the teachings of Dr. Wayne Dyer, my Western guru.

Becoming a Healer

One morning, in massage class, I was giving a massage to a fellow student, Sheila. I scanned her energy path and realized she was in a bad space. Sheila was angry and upset with her mother and sister. She told me she had mentally divorced herself from her family and had not spoken to them for weeks. I searched my mind for a healing tool and thought of a pink quartz crystal that was on my nightstand back at home. Mentally, I visualized the pink crystal transmitting love and pink light directly into the center of her heart. I had energized the pink quartz by placing it outside in my garden at night to absorb the energy of the moon. Silently, I projected sweet emotions of love and forgiveness, speaking silent words into her body, saying, "Forgive, forgive, forgive." Sheila needed to forgive and love so that she would be free from emotions of anger and depression that were unsettling to her entire existence. She was sick and angry and mad at the world.

After we broke for lunch, I returned to class to find the entire student class gathered around Sheila. The sobbing girl came over to hug my neck and thank me for what I had done. She excused herself from class to go tell her mother and sister that she still loved them and was very sorry for her actions. My massage instructor, Mr. Becker, pulled me aside to whisper in my ear that someone in the class was becoming a healer.

My most successful endeavors of healing come to fruition when I give energy from a sacred space of love, nothing more and nothing less and with no expectations of the outcome.

Digest Your Thoughts

> Finally, brothers, whatever things are true, whatever things are honest, whatever things are just, whatever things are pure, whatsoever things are lovely, whatsoever things are of good report; if there be any virtue, and if there be any praise, think on these things.

> — Philippians 4:8 (KJV)

Through many mentors, such as Louise Hay, the admirable, late author of *Healing with Words* and *Empowering Women*, I have learned that our thoughts must be digested as thoroughly as the food we eat. After reading Louise's works, I concluded that healing manifests within the mind, heart, and spirit.

When we sit down to eat a meal with our family, we must focus on warm conversation. If we are reverent and appreciative, the parasympathetic nervous system will kick into gear, delivering precious enzymes for the digestion of food. By offering gratitude, we also form a bond of health, love, and camaraderie with one another. As a friend of mine once said, "Amen, pass the spiritual biscuits and gravy."

Focus on Peace

Think thoughts that bring you joy even if you are worrying about your brother-in-law who has cancer. Change hope to knowing and speak over his healing. Do not talk about what is missing from his healing; profess that he is healed, sing it, and thank God for his healing at least three times a day to declare he is cancer free.

Holistic Modalities

During my internship at Futuristic Health, I became increasingly amazed by the resilience of the human mind and body. I soon discovered that by speaking, feeling, and expecting to be healed, the process of healing is set into motion. This mental preparation allows us to expect positive results.

When we become totally dedicated to our health, we are tipping the scale in our favor. Visualization and joy expedites healing to complete the task of recovery. I strongly urge clients to dismiss any doubt or conflict connected to their desire to heal. "Cancel that" are strong subconscious commands to abolish negative thinking. Positive affirmations will allow you to move into the sweet spot of healing.

In 1998, I received a naturopath certification from the non-accredited Clayton School of Natural Healing. After years of offering nutritional courses to the public, the school was closed. I appreciate the knowledge I acquired on specific herbs, foods, and vitamins. I gleaned an education from this expansive academic facility sponsored by Lloyd Clayton and his family.

The search for an organic solution to health problems initiated a discovery of superior remedies. Such remedies consist of cleanses that target vital organs, most prominently the liver, gallbladder, kidneys, and colon. My naturopathic studies compare and illustrate modalities and treatments that pioneered discoveries from long ago.

Futuristic Health grew from offering massages and foot baths to a full-blown healing facility in the year 2000. Here, I witnessed many healing miracles. My friend Evelyn once said that McVean Clinic was the last-stop clinic before a sick person broke down and went to the hospital. I served incessantly, very often skipping lunch breaks on busy days at the clinic. I have seen patients be dismissed from a liver transplant list, infertile women have babies, kidney stones disappear, insomnia reversed, migraines disappear, and thousands of gallbladders healed.

In 2014, I moved to Ruidoso, New Mexico, to study herbal oils and Native American herbal remedies. I am currently practicing as a health counselor at Benbrook Medical with Rubia Sadiq, MD, in Benbrook, Texas, and the Zen Den Wellness Center in Granbury, Texas

To convert my career change from massage therapist to an alternative health practitioner, I mastered Contact Reflex Analysis (CRA) and attended conferences and seminars all over the United States to accumulate credit hours for my certification. Contact Reflex Analysis was taught by Dr. Dick Versendaal. He invented amazing modalities of acupressure testing and produced instruction manuals with his daughter, Dawn Versendaal Hoezee. In this technique, acupressure points are tested to identify congested organs through the use of kinesiology, i.e., muscle testing. I continue using contact reflex analysis as a muscle testing technique and gauging tool of meridian lines within the body to discover root cause and effect of illness.

Holistic physician Dr. Bradley Nelson, creator of a technique for releasing trapped emotions, states in his book *The Emotion Code,* "Muscle testing can tell us about the overall health and balance of our bodies." I use the client's outstretched arm to indicate weak acupressure points.

These contact points are used to detect anything from yeast infections to kidneys failure. I implement this technique to test clients in office or long distance. Energy is energy—it is here, it is there, it is everywhere. It is our best tool to direct, create, and manifest healing. Since the turn of the century, Futuristic Health has been blessed to serve.

Opening the Can of Worms

During my daily meditations, I became aware of a guiding presence from the Holy Spirit, which seemed to be beating the drum inside of me for answers to questions concerning uncommon causes of illness. Christmas, in the year 2000, I received an encyclopedia on insects and earthly crawling creatures. I opened the book and turned immediately to parasites and their cross contamination into the human species. This startling information was of tremendous value for me as I had not previously considered this fact as a possible cause of illness for people with debilitating diseases. Alarms went off in my head like a code-red alert in an emergency room. I was determined to investigate parasite infestations in sick clients as a leading cause of disease. The probability of infestations would account for low blood volume in people, which could factor in thousands of other debilitating health problems for the entire human race.

Passion for Life

Medical doctors tried to discourage me from having a baby by suggesting I have a hysterectomy at the age of thirty-three. More than one fertility specialist rejected my request for treatments after I presented their office with laparoscopic photographs of my scarred female organs. One Fort Worth group of specialists told me that it would be impossible to have a successful in vitro fertilization. It was now up to God and me. My quest for a college education focused on natural cures to heal the general public and hopefully my infertility. I could not fathom a diagnosis of this nature. I was proud that I could have treatments at my very own healing center, which included massage therapy, nutrition supplementation, foot baths, foot reflexology, and B.E.S.T., bio energetic synchronization, a form of emotional healing. There was no shortage of staff at Futuristic Health who offered to massage points of reproductive organs located on the bottom and sides of my feet. I lavishly massaged those reflex zones applying essential oils with great hopes of reversing the diagnosis of infertility. As I lay on my massage table imagining blue balloons floating on top of my ceiling, I thanked God in advance for restoring my female organs. "Thank you, God. I am healed; I am having my baby." Words of self-encouragement were spoken in faith.

During the initial phase of my practice, it became as clear as Gabriel's trumpet that I could heal myself. I began taking a probiotic three times per day along with liquid kelp to enhance ovulation, and soon my TSH levels began climbind the charts. I was praying it forward for women like myself with infertility problems. I knew the day would come when the one ovary I had remaining as an egg-bearing organ would be enough to make my baby mama dreams come true.

The vision blessing I used for healing seemed to work quite well. I closed my eyes every morning when I woke up and visualized a little scrubbing bubble sliding up and down my one and only fallopian tube. This was the tube that was blocked, or so I was told. I remembered the TV commercial of the little bubbles smiling and sliding around to clean dirt and grime from hard to reach places. The scrubbing bubble was blue and white with a big smile on his face. My mind became so familiar with my little bubble friend that I could just think of his hard work and he would come to my visual aid each time I asked him to restore the scarred tube.

My cousin and I attended a family reunion in Spring Town, Texas. Frances and I began our trip by stopping at the mailbox to mail a letter I had written to God, simply addressed "Heaven." In the heaven letter, I inked soulful expressions of courage to beat my biological clock, asking God for a child. Like a bottle of merlot preserving itself in the cellar of my heart, I was ready to uncork the miracle of life.

Driving out to the reunion, we saw an antique store called the Old Rock House. My eyes couldn't help but notice the sweet little baby cradle displayed on the cluttered front lawn of the store. I teased my cousin, saying I would buy that baby cradle on the way back home. I was happy to see all of my relatives and their children at that summer picnic. In the past I had felt sorry for myself when I saw cousins my age with children. I was certain I had been ignored by the stork that refused to flap his wings for me. I knew I had to impress on my mind a belief that things were changing for the better. I told my folks the next time we had a family reunion I would be there with my very own bundle of joy. I could sense the negative vibrations of those who knew my health problems. To add insult to injury, my husband and I had chosen to go separate ways a few years back and end our marriage due to my infertility diagnosis.

On the way home, Frances and I did stop at the Old Rock House to look at the precious baby cradle. As we pulled into the drive, so did a dark-eyed, young Italian man. He made a U-turn in his brown 280 Z car, stirring up a small dust storm as he whipped into the Rock House parking lot. He hurried up the path where I stood looking at the cradle and politely smiled, asking, "Do you want a boy or a girl?" My heart skipped a beat as I noticed his big smile; thick, wavy hair; and strong body. I snickered, "A boy, why do you ask?"

We did not know the plan the universe and the soul of our unborn child had masterminded for us. As God and all the angels would have it, I gave birth twelve months later to a loving bundle of joy, and he was a baby boy. The light of my life is my twenty-four-old son, Milan Harris Harting.

After years of helping clients restore their personal health, I am honored to share this collection of healing stories to educate the hearts and minds of readers and bring to each of you futuristic health today. May the healing light of God ignite within you and put wings to your prayers.

Baby in Cradle

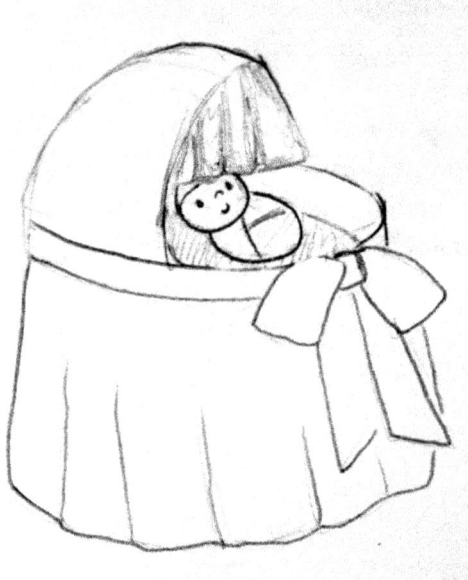

ACKNOWLEDGEMENTS

My clients have given me permission to tell their stories, and I am blessed to have known them, served them, and loved them all. I have changed the names of my clients and the details of their personal lives in order to respect their privacy. Over the past eighteen years, many beautiful women have sat behind the wooden school desk at the office. Some of these office administrators have moved on and perhaps even crossed over the mountain to reside in their spiritual houses of eternal grace. I respectfully take time to acknowledge these dedicated people.

Special Thanks

Esther Fyock, thank you for the six months of editing and creation of the Holy Health. Your praying it forward for the completion of this book has blessed me, and I appreciate and love you. Your dedication to heal the sick truly inspired me throughout every chapter.

Paula Vermillion, my wonderful, compassionate sister who deserves an award for entertaining clients when I was running behind schedule, may your spirit continue to evolve.

Linda Browning, for all of your professional typesetting to complement my brochures and charts. I also appreciate your keen eye for editing the newsletters and much-needed web page. May your spirit shine eternally.

Tammy King, for helping me to set boundaries and for thoroughly understanding the term *organic*.

Frances Freeman, my sweet cousin for taking time out of your busy schedule to travel to the office every Wednesday morning to perform foot reflexology treatments.

Caron Beck, for assisting me with my spinal adjustments and surrogate muscle testing.

Gina Hasley, for your secretarial work, prayers, and dedication to holistic healing.

Glenna Tarvin, for your skills of keen organization and three years of dedication to Futuristic Health.

Tammy and Kevin Watson, bless you for your hard work on setting up my original web page, which is still floating out in cyberspace.

Dr. Dyer, thank you for clear guidance of training the mind to produce miracles. I see the magic. Your guidance and optimism has imperatively directed us to reach for the stars. May your inspirational books continue to guide us as your spirit dwells within our hearts forever.

Dr. Dick Versendaal for all the healing information you shared with me. I am serving humanity in a holistic realm because of you, and I truly loved your sharp humor and analogies for keeping the body tuned up and running like an automobile. May you rest in eternal peace knowing that Contact Reflex Analysis has saved many lives.

Ronnie Williams, my very good childhood friend who encouraged me to continue my path to healing when I felt miserably sick. You had faith that I would heal, and I did. I will always cherish your encouragement and friendship. May your star shine forever.

Thank you, eternal light, for giving me the wisdom, guidance, and power to continue healing the world.

INTRODUCTION

Long ago, the only medicines available to country folks were medicinal plants grown in their garden or wild herbs gathered from the forest. Knowledge of herbal medicine was passed down from generation to generation. Many of these old-fashioned healing treatises are refurbished in *Futuristic Health Today*. The healing modalities presented in this book are unique; unlike conventional healing, the practitioner is encouraged to maintain sweet emotions. Love, forgiveness, thankfulness, and gratitude pave the path to physical and emotional healing. Keep these emotions flowing and collect your ticket to health and happiness.

Thousands of clients have healed themselves by eliminating a trail of poignant thinking. It is true that stressful thoughts create stress hormones, which unfortunately cause deterioration of the body. On the other hand, uplifting thoughts and laughter give your immune system a real boost. Sing to yourself, lull yourself into healing. Speak words that encourage your T cells to defend you and coax them into supporting your immune system. Ask your spirit to stay in harmony with your desires to be well and prepare to heal. If your spirit is lacking contentment, the connection to emotional joy is blocked and will impede healing. Unhealthy individuals are often mentally disconnected from joy. When we change our diet to consume organic plant life and vegetables, we can anticipate positive results and automatically start to feel better. As our search for organic food broadens, so does our focus on the value of health.

If you find yourself on a treadmill in a crowded gym thinking of the negativity you have created in your life, I suggest you zip up your gym bag and go out into nature. Stop at the first sight of a tall oak tree, turn off your car, get out, sit in nature and have a heart-to-heart with God. Here, in the midst of God and nature, I urge you to make an agreement between your body and spirit to live each day with joy and laughter. Work on cleaning your thoughts as diligently as you work on having a beautiful body.

Common Thread

There is a common thread in debilitating health, and this thread is indigestion due to the consumption of foods void of enzymes. *Futuristic Health Today* provides proof that the body is a living organism that responds favorably when given organic food to nourish it. Though the preparation of organic food is time-consuming, I believe it is well worth the investment. You will see an awesome change in your health if you begin adding organic plant protein to your diet. Search for nutritious vegetables, fruits, nuts, and seeds to supplement your daily food intake. Be sure to cook only organic meat and take added enzymes if you eat animal protein. Estrogen-enhanced meat in farm raised chicken and beef is rumored to be a precursor of breast cancer in women as well as men.

Fast food boulevards bombard the hungry in every town, offering quick meals for working parents to serve the family. The world is in a hurry; the soccer mom, the college student, all of us live in a complex society. If you are unable to find time to prepare health food in your own kitchen, order on line convient, ready to make meals at home from Blue apron or Green Chief. You are the backbone of this country—please make it a point to prepare wholesome foods because your health and longevity depends on the next meal you eat. Break the habit that has taken you away from owning health and give yourself time to prepare meals that support life. Give your body what it needs. Processed food tricks the liver and pancreas into a mock run of submitting enzymes. These precious digestive enzymes become dehydrated from chemicals in processed foods.

Our delicate digestive organs cannot compete with food substitutes. Like the little boy who cried wolf one too many times, the digestive system is worn out from asking the body for enzymes to aid in the digestion of inorganic food products. Our bodies cannot live on food that has been microwaved, scalded, frozen, and whipped into a fabulous, perhaps taste-worthy, yet non-nutritious experience. Our taste buds have been temporarily delighted, but the cost is a lack of nutrition, lack of energy, and lack of joy from eating imitation foods. When we start to pull on this common thread, we find a denominator of toxins that are accumulated in the body from the food we eat, the drugs we take, and the thoughts we think.

Pharmaceuticals have a very positive place in modern medicine and have saved many lives, but somewhere in our future, human survival will depend on effective medical alternatives. A depressed person, once he or she has cleaned the liver, might find relief by using phosphatidylserine or hydrophilic CBD oil as an alternative to antidepressants and pain killers. When herbs and food can be used as medicine, the living body will rise to the occasion. Synthetic enzymes and chemicals, dyes and artificial flavorings can no longer be overlooked as easily as MSG was when it first crept into our food chain. The toxins in our blood essentially become the fuel that propels sickness in our bodies.

When I am treating a person for a particular illness, I investigate their eating habits. Many times, it takes several appointments before my client will confess to information that is contributing to his or her illness. For example, a person who is feeling exhausted and has symptoms of swelling and edema might eventually tell me they have been drinking soft drinks or using artificial sugar as a sweetener in his or her morning coffee. In my observations, most diet products such as sugar replacements, though they may be calorie free, contribute to depression and dehydration of organs. If a person must have a fizzy drink, he or she can substitute soda pop with carbonated water served with fresh cut organic oranges or lemons. Chemicals and caramel dyes in soda pops taint the blood and hang out in the adrenals and kidneys, causing edema in the lower back, neck, legs, and feet. Congested kidneys are responsible for a myriad of diseases. Hip replacements, plantar fasciitis, knee replacements, and many crippling diseases are stemmed from kidney stones.

Kidney stones and gallstones manifest quickly when artificial dyes, chemical in dairy and artificial sugars infiltrate our blood. It is your responsibility to be completely honest with yourself concerning which inorganic foods you should eliminate from your diet. You know your poison so begin to confront yourself with the debilitating food choices.

A commonality among clients who find themselves beaten down from a health crisis is the mistake of dwelling on problems. You attract what you think about, what you focus on expands. Being ill and dealing with disease can certainly cause negativity and depression. Likewise, negative emotions can create illness. I have learned that lung problems can originate from grief and kidney problems manifest when a person is angry. Thyroid problems can originate from self-doubt and insecurities, and pancreatic problems arise when life becomes too hectic and void of sweetness.

Futuristic Health Today unveils a merry-go-round of sickness and gives birth to successful healing formulas that will cut straight to the heart of the problem. When put into action, the golden rules, praying it forward, and vision blessings can free you from rabid thoughts, hopelessness, pain, and suffering. If you're looking for a new direction that leads you to a life of longevity, keep reading ... before cancer or worse, death, has crept into your mirror image and slipped an unhealthy noose around your neck.

As you read, take note of the common thread woven into sickness in the human body and consider if it is time to unravel a pattern formed by poor eating habits and unconscious addictions.

Analogy of an Automobile

Dr. Versendaal, DC, CRA, taught classes in chiropractic college and familiarized students with the mechanics of a car. He compared the human body to the body of an automobile: The heart is the motor that must continue to run; the liver is the human filter to screen out toxins; the thyroid is the accelerator that pushes us through the day and night; and the adrenals are a backup to the alternator to kick start the motor.

Automobiles today are run by computers, and comparatively speaking, the brain is an awesome computer that controls the body machine. Sometimes the food we love refuses to love us back. A love of half and half in our coffee may taste wonderful, but our kidneys would appreciate a substitute of coconut or cashew milk instead. One example of an ingredient found in processed food is high fructose corn syrup and other sugar substitutes. We have learned this non-food ingredient actually increases hunger as our bodies are continually searching for purer food to digest. Keep the body machine tuned up, give it the right fuel, and it will run for many years.

Client Responsibility

The decision to seek natural treatment for disease requires a gradual change in what you eat; grabbing celery sticks or apple slices instead of a bag of greasy chips will reward you with enzymes for digestion. This change begins with buying fresh ingredients for making a vegetarian pizza at home instead of ordering yellow cheese pizza with processed pepperoni freshly delivered to your front door. Create good health by forming better habits. Hone in on negative thoughts and stop yourself before you wreck yourself. Life changes are mastered one step at a time, so take the first step that will lead you to a purer, healthier life. Your body is a temple of God. If you backslide on your pilgrimage of restoration, don't beat yourself up. Pat yourself on the back for every good choice you make and move forward by weaving into your life patterns of healthy food to eat. Pack an old-fashioned sack lunch rather slaming down a processed quick fix to calm hunger.

We may be compelled to research a symptom to self-diagnose and treat an ailment by searching on the internet for answers. Not everything we read on the internet is true, nor are the suggested remedies always safe. Sometimes the suggested cure may be a total detriment to our well-being. For example, a client convinced he had microscopic skin parasites went to several doctors who told him he was delusional and treated him for allergies. Taking matters into his own hands, he searched the internet, found a web site about misdiagnosed parasites, joined a chat room, bought products advertised as safe, and continued to self-diagnose while chatting with other people who were experiencing the same problem. When people become desperate for answers, they may latch on to costly mistakes. Please seek alternative health counselors who can assist and monitor you to optimal health.

Our responsibility is to become aware of our bodies' signals. A heartbeat in our necks or ears when we lie down to sleep; nervousness; or a severe headache may be messages from our bodies to pay closer attention. If you begin to experience a negative side effect from a supplement you have taken, it could be a result of your body releasing toxins too quickly. If you suspect you are detoxifying excessively, you may need to take less of the product. Should the side effects continue, it is probably time to discontinue that treatment.

Beloved, let us love one another, for love is of God,
and everyone that loveth is born of God and knoweth
God. He that loveth not, knoweth not God.

— 1 John 4:7–8 (KJV)

Defining God as Creator

When I use God's name, let me make clear that I acknowledge God as the Creator, a unified, conscious, subconscious, and unconscious energy that every human being on this planet has contemplated at some time in his or her life. Many times, a health crisis can stimulate a need for action that is described as a phenomenon, i.e. a healing, a miracle, or the cure to make a person whole again. I have observed when patients are critically ill, they turn to a higher power. When I use the word *God*, I am referring to this higher power. I ask you to give all the glory to God when you are healed. The energy of God has resonated long before the world began, so give the glory of healing to its originator. To define God is too large a task for me, but by focusing on one energy alone, that being love, know you will be drawn closer to a complete definition.

Recipe for Your Miracle

I stopped waiting for the world to give me what
I wanted, I started giving it to myself.

— Byron Katie

For my fifth birthday, I received an Easy-Bake Oven. I was so excited to bake for my father every day to surprise him with delectable, or perhaps not so delectable, cookies when he came home from work. I remember one day he took the cookie and thumped it on the kitchen table. My cookies came out like hockey pucks because I was lacking a recipe to make the perfect cookie for my pops. In each chapter I have listed ingredients for the recipe to prepare your miracle of happiness and supreme health.

Ingredient One: Praying It Forward

My recommendation is simple—a daily routine of prayer,
offered in faith, to enhance health and wellness.

— Mark Stengler, ND, author of *The Natural*
Physician's Healing Therapies

In my years of practice, I have prayed it forward many times for sick clients and discovered the more I prayed for others, the better I felt. I visualize a golden chain of energy as I pray for the sick. I believe the energy of prayer is forming a circle of light as a link to healing. Because requests for healing are offered as an unconditional act of love, healing vibrations are sent into and throughout the entire planet. When a person has lost control of the good life by developing bad habits, we should lift him or her up in prayer. This is what we call praying it forward, the keystone of *Futuristic Health Today*. When we pray it forward, we are summoning the spirit of God by speaking positively for those incapable of pulling themselves out of the realm of sickness. Praying it forward is a powerful application that literally manifest miracles for you and others.

Pray as if your prayers have already been answered and double your blessings. During the day, speak favorably over the people who you know for sure need healing. Joyful words can activate healing very quickly. You are the prayer giver, the one who prays it forward with positive statements. You are the giver of love and you, holy compassionate, are dedicated to giving and receiving healing today. Pray it forward for yourself by speaking answered prayers for someone else. For example, "Thank you, God. Micah is feeling stronger each day and can walk again." Spoken words definitely create reality.

Close your eyes and go into a meditative state where God's promise to heal has already been fulfilled. We are all connected to God's golden chain of healing energy. Change *hope* to *knowing*, trust more, love more, forgive more, and be assured that speaking positive for results will change your life today. If you are blood type B or AB, you are the chosen one to stop the sickness before it spreads. Go deep within your heart and gather compassion for people who need your love and guidance. Your blood type is sensitive to the needs of others. Use your talent to direct healing energy to those you sense will benefit from spoken words of healing. You can generate and initiate energy from a distance. Use praying it forward and let blessings boomerang throughout the day.

Ingredient Two: Golden Rules

As I see it, every day you do one of two things:
build health or produce disease in yourself.

— Adelle Davis

The herbs and supplements described in each chapter are not meant to replace any medicine prescribed by your health-care provider. Be sure to follow relevant directions on product labels and consult your pharmacist or physician before using herbs and natural supplements.

Golden rules lay out guidelines and nutritional therapies for health problems related to Alzheimer's, depression, colon, pinworms, thyroid, kidneys, gallbladder, prostate cancer, digestion, insomnia, and pancreas. Each story has a golden rule section to help you understand which vitamins, herbs, and whole foods are best used for healing these specific problems. Some protocols may sound familiar to those of you with knowledge of vitamins and herbal supplements. You may notice that golden rules are repeated for many of the same health problems because I follow a holistic approach of proper digestion and organ cleanses as major healing tools.

Speak It Real

I have established that thoughts must be digested, so choose words that go down easily. When thoughts are not digested, negativity stagnates in the digestive system, causing undigested food to wreak havoc by leaving a trail of bacteria in the organs and blood. The price to pay is an unsettling disease that can cause gallstones, kidney stones, diabetes, blackouts, infertility, Alzheimer's, and cancer.

I have provided healing remedies that can be purchased from your health food store. Cleanses will benefit you best after recommended nutrition has been taken for a few weeks or even months. The herbs and supplements recommended in *Futuristic Health Today* are suggested to support, cleanse, and purify vital organs. I have seen amazing benefits from organ cleanses; all you need do is follow directions. It doesn't take long for your system to be "all go" after the first, second, or third organ cleanse, depending on your level of toxins. After participating in an organ cleanse, you should not need to continue taking a fistful of supplements on a daily basis. There are only four pathways to release bacteria from your body: lungs, skin, colon, and kidneys. Exercise in moderation, begin dry brushing to cleanse the skin, be sure you have at least one bowel movement a day, and drink plenty of water.

In my nutritional practice, I use several different types of digestive enzymes as well as herbs and vitamin supplements to improve these four pathways. If the client is taking the nutritional protocol that I recommend, I am the second one to know because their testing score will show rapid improvement. I use several formulas of parasite remedies to dry out the amoebas' life force that is often consuming our precious bodily fluids. People who test positive for parasite infections can become anemic and should use chlorophyll or blackstrap molasses and eat leafy greens as well folic acid and B_{12} for blood volume support.

I have noticed that people with the blood Type O are speed healers. They are the heartiest, most resilient human beings on the planet. Type O's are typically lactose intolerant and, unless they can get their heads in the game by eliminating dairy, they have lost the race before the whistle blows. I suspect type O's possess an extra-long common bile duct because this duct will often test as blocked. You can bet if blood type O's are feeling bad, choline, bitter melon, and inositol supplements can put a smile back on their faces.

Ingredient Three: Vision Blessing

We must go beyond the constant clamor of ego, beyond the tools of logic and reason, to the still, calm place within us: the realm of the soul. In the midst of movement and chaos, keep stillness inside of you. Our minds influence the key activity of the brain, which then influences everything: perception, cognition, thoughts and feelings, personal relationships; they're all a projection of you.

— Deepak Chopra

You may be at a busy airport or sitting at your desk during the afternoon. Wherever you are, you can always go to a quiet place in your mind to vision bless yourself. The vision blessings can be completed within a few minutes, as science has documented that subconscious thought travels faster than the speed of light. I have accomplished, with good results, a vision blessing within thirty seconds. You will know when your subconscious switches from hoping to knowing because you will possess a peaceful feeling in your heart. You will feel confident when you open your eyes and return to your normal activities.

The vision blessing is an imaginary mental exercise provided through spirit to help my clients overcome sickness. Negative thoughts can be reversed by visually instructing your brain to believe with hope, faith, and excitement that healing has arrived. Most people dwell on negative situations as a simple means to cope, control, or escape, but negativity creates acid, which is a breeding ground for disease. A vision blessing is fun to imagine and is designed to instruct the right side of the brain to enhance healing. Jose Sylvan, the founder of Sylvan Learning Center, suggests that you visualize the image moving from the left side to the right side of the brain.

When I first opened my office, I used the vision blessing to direct new clients into my office by imagining my appointment book with names in time slots and dates. Steadily, blank spaces began to fill in with new clients. Imagination did turn into reality. You can alter your vision blessing to suit your specific needs. For example, when I wanted to start a family and knew all odds were against me, I would visualize blue balloons on the ceiling or tied to my mailbox. Go to your mental place of healing and shed the worry. Give your vision a feeling of excitement and as you go on about your day imagine what it would feel like to be completely well. Give yourself a couple of at a boys, hip hip hurrays, woopie and high fives. If it is a challenge to stay focused on your vision, gently pick up where you left off. and calmly instruct your mind to focus on the vision blessing for thirty seconds. Worries and the day's to-do list may invariably come into your thoughts, and this is where you smile and say yes. Think of how your thoughts and feelings are shaping reality. By doing so, you will be able to refocus into the vision. The word *yes* is the most the alkalizing word in the English language. Take advice from folks with type A blood; they can crack you up with laughter with their quirky personalities. We depend on their special flare in the arts, music, and comedy.

If anyone can master the vision blessing, it is those who have type A blood. Type A must see, feel, and think themselves into a state of excitement and awareness. If you give them a task to complete, it is best you describe the job with fervor and to perfection. It is important to use the right side of your brain and train yourself to relax during each vision blessing. The final outcome is a magical result that taps into creative healing. You will be amazed at the tremendous decrease in your stress levels by simply performing vision blessing several times a day. Exaggerate the final outcome by giving yourself a feeling of ecstasy.

ALZHEIMER'S:
FORGETTING EDWARD

I met Ed in the year 2000. This was the year of the knight in shining armor. Following a trip to Europe, I became intrigued with the knights in armor standing in the store windows in Amsterdam, the Netherlands, and Venice. I knew immediately the office building I was considering for my practice was the correct choice when I saw the knight standing stoically in the lobby next to the for-rent sign in the office window.

The millennium was also the year my nutritional practice blossomed into a full-blown career. If I were a gardener waiting for my orchids to bloom, I may have given up hope. Very quickly the front and back door of that office building was opening my way. I was nervous about meeting Ed, who came into my office following a diagnosis of Alzheimer's disease. I was sitting at my desk when Ed and his wife came in for an interview. I was a tad bit uncomfortable when we discussed his disease, as he sat straight up in the chair looking confused. I corrected myself for speaking about him in third person. He was obviously hearing me speak but not completely comprehending the necessity of a diet change and a much-needed nutritional protocol.

With each appointment, Ed was more willing to share feelings of crippling anxiety, which by his account kept him emotionally locked down and alienated from society. He spoke with a tone of disgust in his voice as he began to smack his lips and shake his head from side to side, proceeding to explain his feelings of inadequacies when performing simple daily tasks. He shared with me how hard it was for him to hold steady a glass of water. His shaking was too embarrassing to endure.

In spite of his gloomy state, I saw a glimpse of something in his smile that told me he could be lovable and charming. One chilly Monday morning, he came into the office shivering as though icicles were hanging from his hat. I could sense an intense frigidness hovering like a snow cloud in the lobby of my clinic. He had a very sad look on his face. I instructed him to lie down on the table, and I gently laid my right hand on the top of his head and touched a kidney point with my left hand.

I was the battery charger for him today and was proud I had cleared my mind with meditation before his appointment. I could feel fever on his brow, and clearly Ed was experiencing an excessive amount of grief that was stored in his internal organs. I instructed him to think of a particular Christmas when he was young and happy; one that brought him an enormous amount of pleasure, one that completely stood out in his mind. He immediately smiled and told me he had spotted the gift of his first twenty-two rifle. The old man on my table suddenly became a young boy, barely thirteen years of age that cold morning years ago in Midland, Texas. "There it is," he told me, "smack dab under the Christmas tree."

His father had given it to him as a present, and he was pleased as punch just thinking about it. I asked him to take a deep breath, hold his breath in, and expand this memory of happiness and excitement. His muscles and organs began to quiver and shake. As I held his polarity points, providing energy to his organs, I felt a quick jolt of pain enter my right hand. Determined to help him, I began directing the electrical shock to exit into the floor below my therapy table through the bottoms of my feet. The jolt of energy swirled around and around in his body, and I had no choice but to hold my hand steady as electrical impulses kicked like a bull charging from his organs into my hands.

Finally, the unsettled energy calmed down as I held polarity points until I could no longer feel heat or pain in his body. With the help of his Christmas memory and the conviction of my gift from God, he was healed. When he sat up on the table, he began laughing until he cried. I believe he experienced a reemergence of happiness that day in my office, a healing, a shift in his energy. When he stopped crying, he couldn't help but crack a smile as I teased him about the unmatched socks on his feet. After that day, he slowly began to demonstrate joy in his life. I knew I had my work cut out for me; after all, Ed was my first Alzheimer's client. It didn't take many office visits for our hearts to connect.

He willingly participated in my nutritional protocol, except for the days he hid his vitamin pills in the sugar bowl. I saw improvement in his cognizance, and his overall demeanor seemed to be lighter with each treatment he received. Though small in stature, he had machismo and was in every sense of the word a gentleman. I recognized this old soul as a fellow human being who deserved the opportunity to combat Alzheimer's, or at the very least, experience happiness during his course of recovery. His wife and I agreed that we would encourage him to forge the holistic path.

I muscle tested Ed weekly to locate congested organs. I treated him for a congested colon and impacted intestines. I worked his foot reflex points three days a week, and he took ribonucleic acid for control over his shaking and command over his words. This product is more effective when taking ginkgo biloba. The meninges of the brain are three protective membranes coating the skull. Processed sugar can be damaging to this coating so cut back on the sweets as much as possible.

I looked at his chart to see what medicines he was taking and realized my hands were completely tied when it came to discussing his prescriptions. However, I did manage to create a nutritional program that would cleanse his swollen liver and detoxify his colon. Ed had stomach gas from a slow-moving digestive system, so I suggested he begin taking enzymes. Enzymes are an important supplement for people over the age of forty because as the body slows down, so does the digestive system. He enjoyed chewy papaya enzymes because they taste good, and the bonus for him was that they work really fast.

The brain is the body's battery and the fuel this battery uses is protein. It makes perfect sense to begin each day by supplementing the stomach with enzymes to support digestion. If you want to be at the top of your mental game, remember that delivery of digested protein in the blood is the key for the cerebellum to charge the battery. Digestion is an important process for maintaining peak mental health and optimum immune support. Bile distribution must be a daily process to complete the digestion and elimination cycle. When bile is not exported into the stomach via the gallbladder, it is metaphorically speaking as though you shoved your food into a blender and did not turn the appliance on. One or two days of unprocessed food can cause quite a buildup of gas and putrefaction in the stomach. One choline supplement taken each morning was the perfect choice for mental support and digestion.

Ed's liver began to do its job of filtering out impurities and releasing enzymes after he added turmeric and milk thistle to his list of daily herbs. He took the supplement phosphatidylserine to calm nerve cells and support major chemicals that are needed for maintenance of cellular function in the brain.

Our relationship progressed from a professional one to a more familiar and loving one. I never knew either of my grandfathers, and Ed never had children. We filled in a missing piece to a puzzle in our lives. He began to take pleasure in conversations during lunch following his noon office visits. He would speak about the good old days with his faithful dog, Whizzer. He would wait for the brazen Texas sun to fade over the last hill at his ranch in Texas so that he could lie down on the hood of his old pickup truck and count shooting stars. Ed seemed to enjoy storytelling and told those of us who would listen about assisting in the delivery of his prize Charolais calf. "That baby calf was hardheaded," he would say. He loved nature and enjoyed the tiniest of hummingbirds feeding on a salvia bush. He would throw his head back and whistle straight up into the air, launching his happiness into the clouds.

His love of life helped me to slow down a time or two and reconnect with Mother Earth. "Earth to Sherry Dell," I'd say to remind myself to take a few minutes and gaze at wildflowers blowing in the warm wind. I sensed the world was telling me to embrace these gifts that God gave to us, gifts that money could never buy.

One day Ed walked around with a trash can and gathered up scattered trash in the courtyard. I suppose he must have overheard me talking about the windblown trash outside the back entrance to my office. His help was an act of unconditional love, and I recognized a look of affection on his face. As he healed, he began to be aware of the needs of others and reciprocated my caring for him by doing this simple gesture. Give and take, I thought to myself, this truly is unconditional love. I took him shopping for his family one Christmas season, and everything in the entire store was spinning, red, green, silver, and gold. He smiled ear to ear the entire shopping trip.

He took the lead, jetting in and out of aisles, and I held on to his coat so he would not get lost among the crowds. During his final days at Garden Comfort, I hastily drove over to the hospice facility. When I sat down in a chair at the foot of his bed, a Cheshire-cat grin would appear on his face. He gently flipped his feet out from under the bed sheets and stretched them into my awaiting hands for his final foot reflexology treatment. He remembered who I was and what I had done for him; this was all the thanks I ever needed.

Shortly after Edward's soul departed from his body, I saw a vision of him in a dream. He was sitting on an old-fashioned drugstore stool sipping a cup of joe. He was laughing and grinning, telling crazy stories of cattle rustling. Secretly, I believe his soul dwells somewhere in the wild blue yonder, where he hangs his hat on an old fencepost in the Western sky.

Count the days you eat a healthy diet, and those days
will turn into months and years of longevity.

— Sherry Dell

Praying It Forward

We then that are strong ought to bear the infirmities
of the weak, and not to please ourselves.

— Romans 15:1 (KJV)

These words chosen in Praying It Forward were channeled from
my spirit in a meditative state to bring forth healing for you. Feel
free to alter them. Only the Creator knows your needs, and as long
as you are coming from love and willing to give and receive healing,
you are praying it forward.

This prayer of responsibility will fall mainly on the person caring
for the Alzheimer's patient. As laborious and futile as it may seem, I
have personally witnessed that praying it forward for a client's mental
health increases his or her cognitive awareness. Pray with faith as
small as a mustard seed and look for a mountain of results.

Pray: Dear God, I know that my loved one is now able to
remember things. I am delighted that his mental clarity is improving
with each passing day. Thank you, he is happier and has less stress
with every breath he takes. Thank you for giving Alzheimer's patients
hope. Thank you for blessing them with awareness and cognitive
thinking. Thank you for the enzymes and vitamin supplements
that improved my loved one's health today. Thank you for restoring
his happiness and giving him hope for recovery today. He is kinder,
happier, and more understanding each day. Thank you for the days
that I am able to offer complete, unconditional love.

For Caregivers: May blessings be bestowed on you this day. Your kindness and loving support is always appreciated. As you help to support the sick, the entire universe will gladly supports you. You have strength, you have love, and you have knowledge and wisdom when caring for Alzheimer's patients. Say these words over and over to yourself and believe you can make a difference with your service. You offer a gift of stability and love, a characteristic of your own unique self. You offer compassion to all of those whom you care for today. Thank you, thank you, thank you. You are blessed now and forever.

Golden Rules

Health is wholeness and balance, an inner resilience that allows you to meet the demands of living without being overwhelmed.

— Andrew Weil, MD

Herbs and vitamins are not meant to replace any medicine prescribed by your healthcare provider. Be sure to follow relevant directions on product labels and consult your pharmacist or physician before using herbs and natural supplements.

Give Alzheimer's patients enzymes. Make it easy on them by offering chewable enzymes such as Super Papaya Enzyme Plus. Organic apples are a fantastic way to help with digestion because the pectin in the apple is a natural digestive enzyme. Back in the day, there was an adage that stated, "An apple a day keeps the doctor away."

Clean the liver very slowly with phosphorus (orthophosphoric acid). Use twenty drops in water or apple juice. An alternate protocol to drinking apple juice is to take apple pectin pills. This is ideal for those who do not want the added calories from the apple juice or for those who have a sugar intolerance.

Ribonucleic acid (RNA) will help steady shaky hands. It is especially good for the cerebellum, the part of the brain that holds an electrical charge and memory. Phosphatidylserine will calm nerves, support cognition, and aid in overcoming feelings of depression.

If irregularity is an issue, make muffins with bran and use 1/4 t. psyllium husks in the evening as directed on product. Do not over do this fiber, it can build up in the colon. If you are using the psyllium husks and continue to be constipated, stop. One hard and fast rule is to drink the mixture with plenty of water. If the constipation persists, eliminate all powered protein. Drink hot lemon water first thing in the morning followed by a glass of ice water to increase the peristalsis movement in the small and large intestine.

There is evidence that ground flax and chia seeds supply alpha-linolenic acid, which is beneficial for Alzheimer's patients. The digestive tract cannot support healthy fats from the seeds unless they are ground into a fine powder. Studies of this debilitating disease are ongoing, but previous research show evidence that B_{12} is needed to create and maintain nerve cells. B_3, pantothenic acid, and B_9 repair DNA, and B_6 is needed to support chemicals that nerves use to communicate with one another.

I highly recommend taking a very low dose of vitamin D. Half this dose for elderly people, because digesting some is better than none. The supplement vitamin D relaxes nerves and will calm down an anxious patient. One word of caution: this supplement can cause drowsiness if overdosed. Bacopa and sage help to reduce inflammation and protect the brain. Studies on sage show promising evidence that it significantly reduces cholinesterase, an enzyme that contributes to brain damage.

Gotu kola is an excellent herb to help improve memory as it has a healing agent that reduces anxiety and stress. Search health food stores for this loose tea and drink a cup of happiness every day. Cut back on all sugars, desserts, sweet teas, and sodas. Eat organic nectarines, peaches, and pears and use stevia as a sugar replacement. Not all people do well with stevia, I for one have a problem digesting it. One day, during my clinic hours, a very nice elderly couple, Stan and Ella came for their regular appointment. They toted along a nice jar of iced tea to give to me and I was appreciative that hot Texas day. On the way home from the office, I opened the top of the mason jar on the cool drink as I drove home. Around five minutes after I began drinking the tea, I had to pull the jeep over and hold onto my right side. I knew I was having a gallbladder attack. I call the quaint couple and politely asked them what they had used for sweetener in the tea they brought me. After they told me they used stevia, I realized that I must be one of those people who had zero tolerance for the sugar replacement. I use turbinado sugar, the same unbleached crystals I have used for thirty years. Honor your body, just because the nation has touted a newbe food to be a super food does not make it so.

Snack on walnuts, pecans, and sliced almonds. Replace carbohydrates such as cakes, donuts, and pastries with organic cottage cheese wheat toast and sweet organic berries. If you are having a sweet tooth attack, purchase honey with the comb and buy it locally if possible. Spread almond butter on organic rice crackers for a healthy snack. Search for organic almond butter with nothing added. Marathon Food distributes a great tasting almond butter which is available at your local Walmart. Almonds are an alkaline food substance. Try to use this source as a protein substitute. If you choose to eat strawberries, it is imperative to eat organically as the skin on strawberries is delicate and thin and can soak up pesticides. Replace any coffee creamers with almond, rice, or cashew milk or possibly organic soy. All creamer replacements must be organic because the United State is still allowing GMO's genetically modified foods, into our country.

The purpose of substituting is to use an alkaline replacement rather than acid-forming creamers that are scalded or powdered. Substituting milk and creamers with real foods that do not have added enzymes is a health worthy investment that eliminates added chemicals. Remember, digest, digest, digest; this is the key to brain power. Guarantee your mental health by reading labels and searching for the cleanest foods you can afford to buy. Make life fun and interesting for people with this disease. Smile, it is contagious. Always end the day with gratitude.

Vision Blessing: Holy Water

Nothing is softer or more flexible than
water, yet nothing can resist it.

— Lao Tzu

Visualize you are walking out in nature, and as you use your sixth sense, smell the fresh air. Look ahead at the mountains and trees and hear the rhythm of splashing water on smooth rocks. Far in the left corner of your mind's eye, visualize a beautiful pool of water moving from left to the right side of your vision. Here and now, this water is ready to receive your burdens as it awaits the image of you standing in front of the holy water.

Now begin to brush at your shoulders as if to shed a lifetime of worries that have accumulated there. Brush these worries off your shoulders into the pool of healing water. Make this quiet place in your mind, one of serenity and comfort and one that you trust to help you free up all negativity. Continue the brushing until you can see this negativity take the form of gray matter and dust particles. See these particles leaving the outer layer of your body and dissolve into the water. Negative particles disintegrate in the water as the swift current carries them away.

If you are crunched for time, this vision blessing works well in the morning shower. Be sure to see every last negative particle swish down the drain. If your Alzheimer's patient cannot participate with you in this meditation, then by all means brush their shoulders with therapeutic touch and do it for them.

pool of water

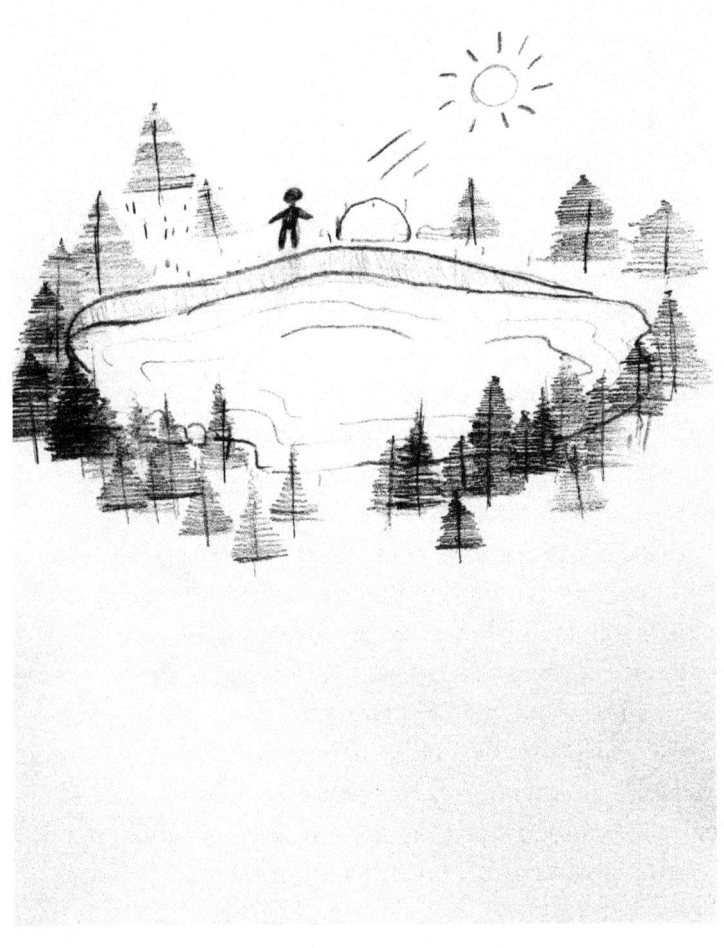

DEPRESSION: WONDERING WANDA

Wanda was a fifty-seven-year-old, unhappy grandma. She was indecisive and uncertain of everything she said. Wanda's daughter, Ann, brought her into the office for treatment for low energy, depression, and lack of motivation. It was obvious that this woman had retreated backstage in the theater of life as she adamantly sat in the rocking chair of gloom. I started asking serious questions as a part of my fact-finding interview before the testing procedure began. Although I should have known by the dull look of her complexion, I asked her what her favorite foods were. Her answer was, "TV dinners, canned soup, or whatever is easiest to fix." Wanda had not eaten fresh foods for many years.

Perhaps TV dinners are common practice for people who don't have time to cook. It is possible they do not have the energy to prepare a healthy meal, mainly because they are eating food that is keeping them drained of energy. I suggested Wanda begin supplementing her diet with whole-food vitamins grown from farmlands by Standard Process. I hoped that she could support her diet with antioxidants and minerals by snacking on brazil nuts, organic berries, and raisins. I shook my head remembering the last client who told me she was having trouble taking her nutritional supplements because she ran out of soda pop. "Dear Lord, how did I get this job?" It is not easy telling people they are wrecking their health by eating frozen meals preserved with chemicals or drinking sodas. In my years of practice,

I have discovered that food is a touchy subject, but I acknowledge the theory of "you are what you eat."

Joy and happiness had become a foreign emotion to Wanda, though her daughter told me her mother was once a happy, vibrant lady. I knew Wanda was experiencing foggy brain from consuming food that had extremely low vibrations. The sweet lady must begin to see the light, I thought to myself. Offering compassion was my greatest asset as a healer, so I began praying it forward for her health. I would speak over her healing in my prayers, and she began feeling positive results as time went by. I recalled my childhood days in church when I cringed and ached when I saw Ms. Thompson's noseless face. It was my job to heal the sick, and I would continue to take my work seriously.

I tested Wanda's brain reflexes and found low numbers on the cortex, the conscious thinking machine. Her spinal fluid was also lacking volume. This fluid is responsible for electrical impulses that support brain activity. Electrolytes increase the volume of spinal fluid, so I sent Ann to the health-food store to buy her mother a powdered electrolyte supplement. One of my favorite supplements for increasing spinal fluid is Cal-Amo. Supplementing with electrolytes is the first step to correcting depression.

As I sat looking at her squirming in her chair, I wondered what could have happened to her to make her aura feel so dense. I was tapping into a grievous feeling of regret that posted on her face. This low vibrational emotion was one she probably visited frequently. It was obvious she was still dealing with a sorrowful tragedy. I asked her if she had been responsible for a loved one, perhaps a family member, a child, or a friend. I could feel an urgency about a closeness that was misplaced or misdirected. Wanda gasped—it was obvious that I had hit the nail on the head.

She told me her husband could not remember who she was. "Dementia," she said slowly and then looked down at her feet as if to sink even lower into a darkness that was consuming her. I quickly stood up and walked around her body, scooping away at her aura with both of my hands. I could see and feel thick globs of green goo coming off her energy field with my hands as I cleared and clean her etheric energy. I instantly felt her denseness clearing and growing lighter as I preformed therapeutic touch on her shoulders. Therapeutic touch was discovered by Dora Kunz, a gifted energy healer, and Delores Krieger, PhD, RN, professor emeritus of nursing at New York University. Years ago, these two ladies developed and standardized the technique and used it to calm down wounded soldiers.

Using my hands, I brushed, combed, and swept away invisible darkness and sadness from my client's energy field. I sensed a heaviness leaving the office as I used therapeutic touch to sweep away old frequencies of disappointment, regret, and solitude. Memories can be a good thing or a bad thing; I encouraged Wanda to think only of the good memories she had mistakenly left behind when her husband fell ill. When she was feeling lonely, she must think of the fun trips, family outings, picnics, and wonderful times she enjoyed when her husband was still active and well. Our memory can bring us fantastic healing when we reminisce the happiness and joys of life. You must find happiness throughout your day. The best way to keep in touch with the emotions of joy is to eliminate criticism and judgement. Dissolving these two bad habits opens up your space to joy and laughter and ultimately healing.

People engage in internal dialogue every day. Choosing positive dialogue can give us euphoric energy. Positive expectations to heal can and will heal us and is a useful tool. I encouraged Wanda to speak favorably about her returning to a life of joy. I also encouraged her to communicate with the plants and flowers in her garden. Plants and vegetables, herbs and animals, trees and rocks, fish and birds are vibrations of God's creativity.

Try this test at home: Choose a piece of furniture that could use some tender love and care, polish it, laugh around it, feel joyful energy entering it, and before long, your entire house will begin to sparkle. Everything has a form of energy that gives it character and personality. Give to yourself inspirational thoughts and manifest healing vibrations to carry you through the day. Fill your house with love and laughter and it will give back to you the same.

Wanda was taking prescription pain pills for lower back pain. Lower back pain is generally caused from impaction of the small or large intestine, kidney stones, or both. Pain pills cause dehydration in the colon, which can make constipation worse. A habit of taking pain pills can cause a never-ending battle of pain and constipation. It is mandatory to maintain a clean, healthy colon for maintenance of interstitial fluids. These fluids saturate and supply nerves and neurons to spark electrical impulses. Enzymes and stomach juices must be present in the stomach for proper digestion to produce adequate elimination. I muscle tested her and suggested she take a stool softener. The muscle test informed her of the approximate dosage she could take at night to ensure perfect bowel movements each morning. A good bowel movement is like winning the health lotto daily. Stool softeners in the form of Senna leaves and cascara sagrada are a winning ticket for this occasion.

The second visit Wanda made to my office was a miracle in motion. Wanda looked like she had invited the sun to shine in her life. She explained to me that the stool softeners I gave her were working like magic. With a smile, she enthusiastically told me she was experiencing more energy and felt like doing things around the house again. You guessed it—she started preparing nutritious meals. Wanda slowly weaned herself off of prescription drugs and antidepressants. I suspected the depression had started from an emotional low when she could no longer identify herself as a loving wife because her husband did not recognize her. The domino effect from her negative thinking impeded her ability to digest food and thoughts, all of which was contributing to constipation. As she walked out of the office door, I bowed my head and thanked God for her quick recovery. I prayed forward her ability to continue taking responsibility for her health.

When you go walk outside, smile and say hi to your neighbor, you are saying hello to an extension of yourself.

— Sherry Dell

Praying It Forward

If thy whole body therefore be full of light, having no part dark, the whole shall be full of light, as when the bright shining of a candle doth give thee light.

— Luke 11:36 (NIV)

These words chosen in Praying It Forward were channeled from my spirit in a meditative state to bring forth healing for you. Feel free to alter them as only God knows your needs. As long as you are coming from love and willing to give and receive healing, you are praying it forward.

Ann's prayer for her mother was, "Thank you, God, for giving me back the vibrant, healthy woman who raised me. My mother has friends who help her enjoy her retirement. She is eating clean, healthy meals. My mother is taking nutritional supplements to heal her body. Laughter and love live in Mom's heart. Thank you, God. Mother is happily counting her blessings every day. She walks outside into her garden and enjoys the sunshine on her face."

Wanda's prayer was easy and simple, and she prayed the same prayer daily. "I am healed, I am whole, I have fun with my friends. My life and family is important to me, and my health comes first." My continued prayer is, asking the divine Creator to fill the hearts of depressed people with love and light to grow their garden of happiness.

Golden Rules

We are indeed much more than what we eat, but what we eat can nevertheless help us to be much more than what we are.

— Adelle Davis

Herbs are not meant to replace any medicine prescribed by your healthcare provider. Be sure to follow relevant directions on product labels and consult your pharmacist or physician before using herbs and natural supplements.

Eat plant protein, nuts, and vegetables for one week, follow this plan, and stick to alkaline-based vegetables. Indulge in organic salads, peppers, beets, greens, walnuts, pecans, fruits, figs, cucumbers, and kiwi. If you're hungry for carbohydrates, sample Dave's Powerseed bread. Wrap this bread in chopped garlic cloves and eat this to help produce enzymes and destroy parasite eggs that may be living in your intestines. The bread is sweetened with fruit juice instead of sugar. Eat foods the color of the rainbow and mix and match steamed vegetables seasoned with garlic, turmeric, ground pepper, rice, and Himalayan sea salt. Nothing is better than cooked pinto beans seasoned with green onions and chopped tomatoes as organic relish.

Substitute ready-made cornmeal mixes with Bob's Red Mill organic cornmeal and stir up some old-fashioned cornbread using almond milk for a milk substitute. Watch for labels on condiments such as ketchup and mayonnaise because there is more sugar and chemicals in these types of kitchen condiments than you could ever imagine. Be sure to bring your reading glasses to the grocery market to read labels on foods and eliminate sugar and corn syrup as much as possible. Enlighten your mental taste buds with a dose of reality. All things that taste good are not good for you.

Make this a week of healing to elevate mental and spiritual health. In weeks to follow, add organic chicken and wild-caught

Alaskan salmon to your diet and switch from plant protein to animal protein. Use all organic protein sparingly. Eliminate ice cream, cookies, and sweets from your diet. Take note that that ice cream unless organic has more chemicals that carter has liver pills. Eat only foods that do not have preservatives or processed chemicals in them. Bake cookies from scratch by using organic flour and unprocessed sugar. Take the vitamin choline to clean out the bile ducts. Indulge in the liver cleanse every year. I do the liver cleanse two weeks before Thanksgiving. This tradition reminds me to give thanks for having a clean, healthy digestive tract. Use a natural laxative and stool softener if necessary. If you are taking pain medication, try supplementing with arnica sublingual tablets and white willow bark. Use the herb bacopa for brain stimulation and take a few drops of Ashwagandha for a subtle dose of tranquility. Don't forget to pray it forward because there is always another person in need of comfort who could use positive vibrations set their way.

Vision Blessing: Rainbow Writing

When you find the courage to listen to your intuition,
step off the familiar path and explore the unknown,
you will be following the calling of your soul.

— Colette Baron Reid

Create a mental vision by imagining you are sitting on a white cloud with a rainbow attached to the left side of the cloud. The cloud can hold the image of your spiritual body as you inhale and exhale ten long, deep breaths. Relax here in the ethers of your mind. Use your finger to write positive words of love, hope, and wellness in the sky. Using the color pink, write "I am love." Use your pointer finger to write the words "I am happy" in blue letters. Next write "I am healed" in yellow and golden tones.

Use the rainbow writing to scroll positive affirmations across the sky by affirming what you desire. Search your imagination for concise affirmations. You can use this vision blessing to write for your wellness and for others. You should use orange and red to uplift your spirits and clearing your mind of discouraging thoughts. If you have a recurring fearful thought, replace it with the opposite polarity when rainbow writing. Example: if you are afraid or use the word afraid during the day, praise god that you're safe and protected. Don't forget to feel safe and secure as you repeat the mantra.

Write these words in a calming violet color scrolling across the sky: "I overcome obstacles, I am safe, and I am blessed with guardian angels today." When you feel content, return to your earthly chair and thank the vision blessing for assisting you with your desires. Use rainbow writing for others to eliminate their insecurities and pray they overcome life's obstacles.

Rainbow

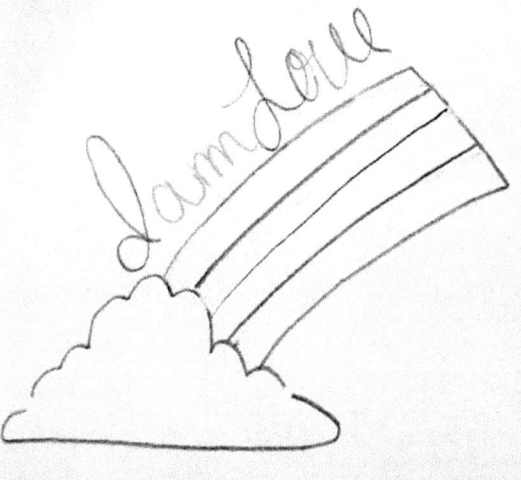

COLON IBS: DEVON'S CLIMB

Devon was a God-fearing, forty-six-year-old man who enjoyed his career as an outfitter. He had a strong physique and lived for hunting and camping in the wilderness. When he gazed down at my desk, I struggled to keep my eyes from staring at the bear claw wrapped in leather neatly displayed on his keychain. He saw me glance at it and told me he had taken the brown bear down in Wyoming.

During the time that I met Devon, he was under tremendous pressure. He explained to me that he had been experiencing colon issues resulting in severe and painful diarrhea that left him feeling weak, fatigued, and dehydrated. I immediately suspected he had contracted a parasite infestation. I asked Devon if he drank water from a stream or river in the mountains when during hunting expeditions. He glared at me, which confirmed that he was not the type who preferred hotel accommodations. "Absolutely!" he said.

He reached inside his blue jean pocket and pulled out a medicine bottle. He told me that his gastrointestinal doctor had prescribed him a strong medicine that was not helping him relieve his gas pain or unexpected bathroom urgencies. Furthermore, his physician had warned him that if his bowels did not calm down with the use of this medicine, the next step in curing his irritable bowel syndrome would be the removal of his small intestine.

What a predicament—a strong and healthy hunk of a man facing surgery that would change his world forever. I sensed his tension as tears streamed down his face, and he flatly told me he

21

could not live with a colostomy. I said, "I like the way you are thinking." He was on board for any alternative approach to healing his irritable bowel disease that I could offer.

As I sat on my swivel chair, I began to sense a feeling of sadness. I saw distant colors of red, black, and orange, which usually inform me of anger and unforgiveness. I could hear his voice go faint in the distance as I started to feel my body become lighter. My head was spinning as I recalled a familiar feeling that reminded me that before the body can heal, the subconscious must release old wounds.

I knew that Devon's medical problem would disappear if he could find a way to release, relax, let go, and let God. I stammered a bit but got back on track as he finished telling me the nature of his symptoms. I detected an invisible swirling heat and pressure in my head, which told me that Devon, like most people, had experienced a tragedy in his life. I asked him if he had lost someone close to him. He questioned me like a detective about how I could possibly know what had happened to him. Amazingly, he even asked me if I believed in God. I told him that it was God who gave me the gift of detecting mental and physical maladies.

We both prayed that day in my office, and he confided in me the story of how he had lost his wife and children tragically some ten years ago. This was truly tragic, and I understood why his immune system was seriously run down. Before our session was over, we were both crying but in agreement that forgiveness was in every sense of the word a beginning to the emotional healing he so desperately needed. I suggested he say or sing words of forgiveness and keep the energy moving through him, so he could accomplish a clearing within a cellular level.

Positive thoughts create energy that defuse subconscious debris. My instructions for him (and for anyone who has suffered a tragic loss) was to keep positive, happy thoughts flowing amidst his soul. Devon questioned me like he was a member of NCIS every time he walked into my office and soon, he became one of my regular clients. We had amazing results once he began to use God's bitter herbs. These herbs dry out any foreign amoebas and bacteria that have settled into the colon. One note of caution: bitter herbs may slightly increase hypertension. Use sound judgment when taking herbs and use muscle testing to aid with dosing. Remember that song and laughter is a fast way to clear away negative energies from the etheric body.

Devon was unable to decide if he contracted the parasites by drinking from contaminated streams or from the wild game that he had caught and eaten. All the same, he had the symptoms of an acute parasitic infestation and was willing to take bitter herbs to clean them from his colon slowly but surely. I was beginning to feel tightness in and around my stomach and was quite sure that I was feeling Devon's gastritis. *This is no fun,* I thought to myself as I begin to repeat the words "I am a righteous child of God." I suggested that he repeat those same words first thing in the morning and last thing at night. I knew if the body was relating to sadness, the only way to reverse it was to fill the soul with joy. From that day forth, I prescribed the words "I am a righteous child of God" like an MD prescribes medicine to their patients. Bacteria leaves the body and alkaline thoughts are invited in when the spirit greets harmony with the righteousness of our soul.

The human body is very resilient. Sometimes, after a few weeks of chronic diarrhea, caused from a parasite infection, the body will adapt to these symptoms and only demonstrate occasional colon problems during the new and full moon. The phases of the moon are when parasites hatch their eggs; the cycle of proliferation repeats itself unless infection can be purged from the body. Bitter herbs, raw garlic, and alkaline foods should be eaten for six months to be sure the last of the parasites' eggs have deteriorated. It is obvious to those infected that their health is declining because they display a gaunt facial appearance and their energy begins to plummet. Headaches, upset stomachs, irritable bowel syndrome, or constipation impedes normal daily activities. Life becomes a grueling process just to make it through each day without embarrassing incontinence. Crawling sensations on the head, skin, and nose will resemble allergic reactions and sleep can be difficult. Skin breakouts resembling eczema are not uncommon as a symptom of a parasite infection. The skin will take control and try to flush out toxins and though we humans only hold a gallon or so of precious blood, the parasites soak it through their skin. Imagine little sponges hatching and absorbing fluid to survive. This is exactly what happens with a parasite infection. The person with the infection will feel dehydrated and begin to bloat in the stomach. When the infection is peeking, their skin will demonstrate red rashes from blood rising to the surface of our skin. When there is not enough of the blood, it stays in the superficial stages just below the surface of our skin, rather than medial or deep when it should be.

Devon does not go outfitting without a travel kit of preventive medicine next to his sleeping bag. In his kit, he carries grapefruit seed extract to correct any stomach issues, bitter herbs, just in case he has contacted parasites, and molasses to help with his iron consumption. He has found solace and peace in his heart over situations he cannot control. He continues to hike and hunt in the wilderness, where he assures me, sitting next to a campfire in the mountains, is like holding hands with God.

Health is something we cannot live without;
forgiveness and love help us to maintain it.

— Sherry Dell

Praying It Forward

Look, there on the mountains, the feet of one who brings good news, who proclaims peace! Celebrate your festivals, Judah, and fulfill your vows. No more will the wicked invade you; they will be completely destroyed.

— Nahum 1:15 (NIV)

These words chosen in Praying It Forward were channeled from my spirit in a meditative state to bring forth healing for you. Feel free to alter them as only the Creator knows your needs. As long as you are coming from love and willing to give and receive healing, you are praying it forward.

Speaking words of blessing and healing will guarantee you a speedy recovery. Simply pray: Thank you, Creator, for directing me to natural remedies that heal my body. I am healed, I am well. Today I have the health and stamina of a young child. I am a righteous child of God." Be aware of your words when you speak about yourself and others. If you have negative opinions about anything, keep it on the down low. I promise you that you will have more energy and stress less if you go to a better feeling place.

May blessings come to those in need of clean food and water. I offer thoughts of clearning and cleaning impure food and water for countries in our Nation. Thank you, spirit for opening the minds of allopathic doctors. Thank you, spirit for healing someone today. I am blessed with the confidence that I am well this very day, this very hour as minutes go be, I am healed. I project healing love and light into the planet.

Today, I am reversing negative thoughts. I am anxious about nothing. I claim ultimate healing minute by minute, hour by hour, day by day. I am confident that I am healed.

Golden Rules

Turn away from the things you don't love and
don't give them any feeling, because they are fine
as they are, they have no place in your life.

— Rhonda Byrne

Herbs and vitamins are not meant to replace any medicine prescribed by your healthcare provider. Be sure to follow relevant directions on product labels and consult your pharmacist or physician before using herbs and natural supplements.

I instructed Devon to take the bitter herbs wormwood, clove, gentian and black walnut to kill off the parasite infection. I also suggested he begin taking a strong probiotic to combat the bacteria in his colon. The hardest part of combating an amoeba infection is trying to convert a daily diet to alkaline-based meals. Take one teaspoon baking soda in a half cup of lemon water five days of each month. The soda will help alkalize your blood, but do not take it any longer than five days.

Check out examples of alkaline food at the end of the book. L-cysteine is the one sure bet that the tapeworm eggs will not survive a life cycle of 120 days. Eat organic eggs and seed bread sweetened with fruit juices for a hearty breakfast. If you are traveling, pack a jar of organic almond butter and seed bread for a protein meal on the go.

Be sure to keep plastic water bottles out of the sun so that you are not drinking chemicals that have seeped back into the water from flimsy plastic bottles. You can actually see the grade of bottle that is imprinted on the bottom of plastic bottles. If the number 1 PETE is imprinted on the bottle, it means that the bottle does not contain BPA but cannot be refilled and is only intended for a one-time consumption. Investigate the numbers on each bottle of water and decide for yourself which plastic bottle to use, if any. Be aware that some chemicals used in plastic bottles can cause cancer. The numbers seven, three, and six are known to be a toxic plastic while one, two, four, and five are somewhat safer.

The perfect drinking container is a glass container or stainless-steel water bottle.

Enzymes, bitter herbs, and probiotics immediately gave Devon relief from gas and stomach pain. As mentioned earlier symptoms of parasite infections can be skin lesions and pimple-like sores on the body. Sometimes the face, neck, shoulders, and arms will begin to itch and break out with pus-filled skin irritations that resembles psoriasis. Adult onset acne is a telltale sign that a person could have intestinal parasites.

If skin lesions do appear, it is a sign that the skin, which is our largest organ, is filtering out impurities. Use the herb yellow dock as a blood builder and add liquid chlorophyll to cleanse and purify the blood. If hands and feet are cold and going numb, reach for a gentle iron supplement. One word of caution: cancer patients should not take iron supplements. Instead supplement the diet with organic spinach, pinto beans, molasses, and bone broth to build bone marrow and hermetic blood volume.

Over 75 percent of my clients presenting IBS and chronic fatigue have contracted intestinal parasites. It is imperative to continue a parasite cleanse for six months. If only one egg is lingering in the intestine, it can perpetuate a vicious cycle of infections for many, many years.

I have seen my clients' emotions spiral out of control when they realize they have parasites living inside of their bodies. Parasites thrive well in an acidic environment. Praying it forward is an excellent tool to calm the emotions and change an acid pH into one of alkaline. Stay calm and be assured that these parasites will not live in a body that is alkaline. Refer to the list of alkaline foods and choose at least three to eat every day. I eat kiwi, avocado, figs, and cucumbers every day. Just like the ocean tides, parasites ebb and flow with the new and full moon. Remember the waning and waxing of the moon will increase the parasite infestation. Be sure not to skip a dose of a parasite cleanse during extreme phases of the moon. In Mexico, the black seeds of a papaya fruit are eaten to kill parasites.

Pray over your food and bless it with white light before you begin eating. Practice love, for it is the highest path to healing. Set an intention to give love to those who are hardest to give love to because they need it most.

Drink three or four drops of grapefruit seed extract (GSE) in water after a meal of fish or any crustaceans. GSE is also a fabulous way to put an end to upset stomachs and viral infections. If you see white grainy seeds that look like rice in your toilet after a parasite cleanse, it is most likely parasite eggs. The same with a substance that is brown and resembles coffee grounds. The appearance of either of these in your toilet after a bowel movement and parasite cleanse is a positive sign you are purging the worms.

The herbs cayenne pepper, thyme, and rosemary will aid in drying out the protozoa. Use it and all bitter herbs with caution. I advise you to take all bitter herbs no more than three weeks consecutively, allowing three to five days off before returning to the protocol. Three weeks on and five days off will keep your body from becoming overexposed or immune to the herbs. Start out in small doses and be cognizant of how your body responds to herbal healing.

Speak words of healing always and do not claim the parasites or give them an ounce of energy. Make positive statements over your healing and be clear and concise with your intentions.

A righteous child of God is a person who has the same consideration for another as they have for themselves.

— Sherry Dell

Vision Blessing: Mountain Climbing

The great Spirit is in all things: he is in the air we breathe. The Great Spirit is our Father, but the Earth is our Mother. She nourishes us; that which we put into the ground she returns to us.

— Words of Big Thunder (Bedagl) Wabanaki, Algonquin

Find a quiet place to imagine you are effortlessly hiking a trail that takes you up to a mountaintop. Visualize green meadows outlining the terrain as you climb to the summit. Once you arrive, remove your shoes. Stand here in this high mountain meadow and breathe in ten deep breaths to receive strength from the majesty. Ask it to empower you through the soles of your feet to the top of your head. Trust that God is healing the sick, driving out darkness and all negativity. Smile and extend your hands up over your head as a motion of victory. Stay here on the mountain and take several extra breaths, inhaling and exhaling negativity. Ask the mountain to bless your body and offer thanks for a miraculous miracle of healing.

path leading to mountain. with a man on top.

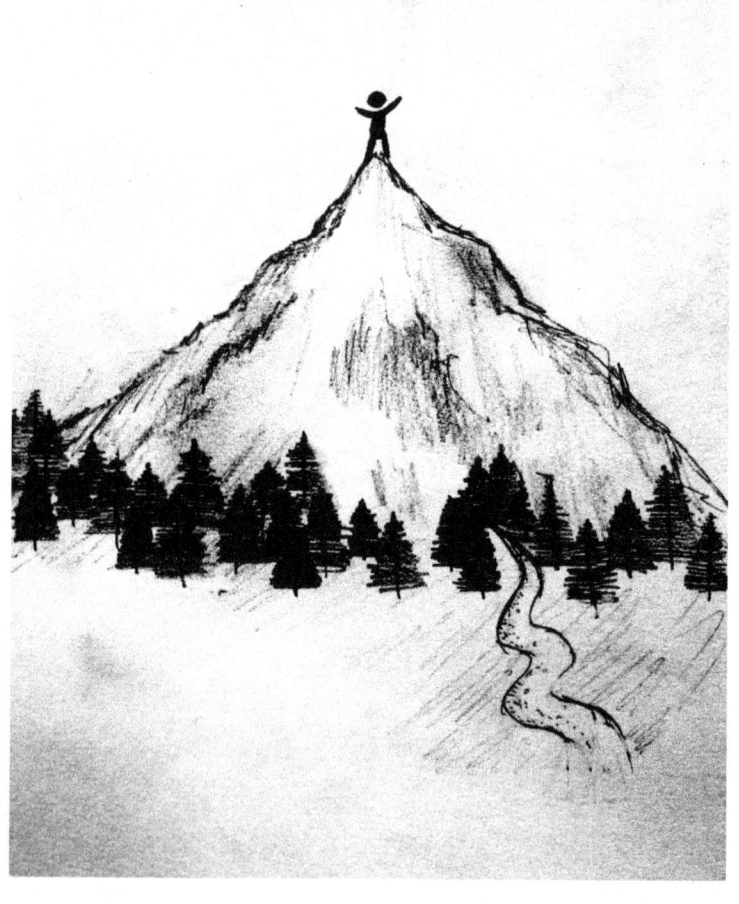

PARASITES: GINGER'S AFFLICTION

A popular elementary school would not permit a five-year-old girl named Ginger to enroll in preschool because she had an inflamed bald spot on the left side of her head. Her mother would pin the hair up and over the girl's head to cover the unsightly sore. Ginger scratched and pick at her inflamed scalp as she whined at the possibility of missing a chance to go to school. The circumference of the bald spot was about the size of an orange that could not be overlooked by the preschool nurse. The child's mother brought her into the Futuristic Health office to see if I could solve the problem. Three pediatricians had prescribed medicines and topical ointments that did not stop the irritation or help with the regrowth of the pretty girl's hair.

When her mother confirmed that Ginger was having constipation problems, this aroused my suspicions. I instinctively knew that the missing hair was due to a pinworm infection. The symptomatic scalp was not contagious but looked to be so. Ginger was willing to take the nutritional supplements I recommended. I was flattered that she trusted me, and secretly I wished that all of my clients, young and old, had the heart of this five-year-old child. We had to work fast; it was spring in Texas, and school would begin in late summer.

As we sat and laughed in my consultation room, I begin to see a vision of Ginger playing outside with her dog. She was wearing a purple cotton t-shirt and a tiny swimsuit. I asked the mother if her little girl had been playing in a sandbox or perhaps making mud pies. The answer was yes to both. I did not hesitate to ask if Ginger had also been experiencing difficulty in having bowel movements. A pinworm infection (*Enterobius vermicularis*) will cause a skin rash, itchy head, yeast infections, thinning hair, and small, goat pellet stool. These amoebas are inhaled through the nose and mouth in the form of microscopic eggs that have been hatched in dirt and sand. The pinworms make their way into the intestine, where they enter the colon and rectum.

There, they soak up precious moisture that causes itching and dry patches of the skin. The itchy skin, nose, head, and buttocks are all due to the parasite sponging up bodily fluids. This parasite mimics allergies and often causes aggravating symptoms to their host for a lifetime. I treat adults for this allergy who most likely contracted this single-cell amoeba from childhood activities or day-cares where the infection is spread. People suffering with pinworms will display irritability, hyperactivity, epidermal irritations, insomnia, tiredness, sometimes lung issues or shortness of breath, grinding of the teeth at night and constipation. Quite a lot of problems from such a tiny pinworm. The real problem is that they lay massive amounts of eggs and are extremely hard to extinguish.

If an infant shows signs of a red body rash, it is most likely a pinworm infection contracted while in the hospital. Prescription creams or topical ointments do not chase the rash away. Use caution when treating infants and contact your local holistic practitioner for guidance and confirmation of this parasite.

Adults can contract this infection from their children simply by holding their hands, kissing, and hugging them. This is why it is so important to check your child's stool for constipation and listen while they are sleeping to hear if they are grinding their teeth at night. You will know when to begin treatment.

Daycare centers and nursing homes are breeding grounds for pinworm infections due to playrooms and crowded sleeping quarters. If untreated, this pesky infection can result in the loss of blood volume that can results in numbness of hands and feet, low back pain, and intermittent dizziness in children and adults. A child or adult may experience irritability and restlessness when this infection is acute.

In just two weeks, Ginger's long red hair began to thicken and grow back on the top of her cute little head. I administered her final checkup before she was allowed to enroll in preschool. Her mother brought her in for a follow-up during winter break, and Ginger was still growing a thick head of red hair, and she was clear of pinworms.

We must teach our children a thousand ways to stay healthy. The survival of our planet depends on their knowledge; they are the future.

— Sherry Dell

Praying It Forward

Now Faith is the substance of things hoped for, the evidence of things not seen.

— Hebrews 11:1 (KJV)

These words chosen in Praying It Forward were channeled from my spirit in a meditative state to bring forth healing for you. Feel free to alter them as only the Creator knows your needs. As long as you are coming from love and willing to give and receive healing, you are praying it forward.

My prayer for all God's children across the globe is to combat parasite infections and stamp them out before the epidemic spirals out of control. I am happy that parents of children have read this information and are taking action to treat any suspicious symptom of a parasite infection. Isn't it wonderful that children diagnosed with ADHD and leukemia are improving by participating in these parasite cleanses? Parents are becoming aware that diet and nutritional remedies can make a weak child strong again. Glorious, unfathomable energy of light, I thank you for the enlightened individuals who aspire to find simple answers to difficult health problems. Thank you, Creator, for the many blessings you have given us. We are educating our children and their children with futuristic health today.

Golden Rules

This is a new day I begin anew and claim and
create all that is good and so it is.

— Louise Hay

The following described herbs are not meant to replace any medicine prescribed by your healthcare provider. Be sure to follow relevant directions on product labels and consult your pharmacist or physician before using herbs and natural supplements.

A pinworm infection is located in the colon and rectum. The pinworm can pass through the intestinal wall and travel into the bloodstream, where they mimic sponges and soak up interstitial fluids and precious blood. Sugar and cokes can be a stimulate for pinworms to increase in numbers.

Symptoms of an infestation can be a blue circle around the mouth; red, itchy rash on the face, arms, and legs; as well as thinning hair in children and adults. The infected person may experience sensations on the skin and grinding of their teeth during sleep. Youngsters rejuvenate themselves by wiggling and moving continuously to keep their bodies and brains active. This activity can cause a weary teacher to suspect hyperactivity and attention deficit problems. Children also pick their noses, eat their boogers, and scratch their heads. This infection is a tough one to combat; a pediatrician may prescribe the drug ivermectin for your child if he or she believes your child has a pinworm infection.

Japan discovered this drug in the late 1970s as a derivative of avermectin. The Kitasato Institute in Tokyo, Japan, has had an immeasurably beneficial impact in improving the lives and welfare of billions of people throughout the world. Originally used as a veterinary drug, it kills a wide range of internal and external parasites in commercial livestock and pets.

Keep some type of exterminating treatment going if the child is displaying any of these signs. The pinworm will lay eggs that thrive in head lettuce, dirt, and sand. Clean all veggies and lettuce with a pinch of baking soda and 1/4 tsp vinegar in water leaving vegetable to soak about five minutes. Rinse thoroughly and spin dry. Sugar exacerbates this problem, so stick to fruit sugar and monitor what your child is eating if you can! My son had a horrible reaction to gummy bears when he was twelve years old. We ended up in the emergency room, and the doctors looked at me as if I were a nutcase when I told them he had a wad of gummy bears blocking his large intestine. Train your child to understand what is good for them and what will make them sick. Wash your hand, wash your children's hands, and check to see if they bite their nails, a true sign of parasites.

My mother told me that her parents wormed her and her siblings during the full moon at the same time they wormed the cattle. The product they used to kill the pinworms was a teaspoon of turpentine in a tablespoon of sugar. This process would attract the worms with the sugar and kill them with the poison, though I don't recommend it because turpentine is not safe for human consumption.

Ginger's story is important to remember because your child or grandchild may exhibit similar symptoms that could cause him or her to be labeled hyperactive. A toddler can be treated with fig powder mixed in applesauce or a few small drops of apple cider vinegar mixed in with their apple juice. Toddlers will pick and pull at their bottoms because the pinworm itches. Children should eat pickles and pickled vegetables to help dry the infection our. Feed a constipated child organic red and green grapes to activate bowel movements. This will purge the pinworms. If you can persuade your child to drink one half teaspoon of vinegar and honey in one half cup water, it will start the deterioration of intestinal pinworms quickly.

Reese's Pinworm Medicine is an over the counter medicine that has instructions for treating children with pinworms age two and older. You may need to buy a few bottles before you have destroyed the last pinworm egg, but it is better than having your child be prescribed the drug Adderall. Pinworm eggs can survive for two to three months, not quite as long as tapeworm eggs. The key to eradicating a parasite infection is to treat it on and off for two to six months straight. Change bedsheets every other night and be sure the child has a new pair of underwear to wear when going to bed. The pinworm prefers to lay its eggs in dry places like sheets and underwear.

Adults and children can use bitter melon, gentian, X-Worm, or wormwood liquid in consistent and conservative doses. I generally use the rule of thumb that two drops of herbal remedies are used per ten pounds body weight. Use organic grain as roughage and if necessary add psyllium husks to almond milk for a nightcap. Eat brown rice or oatmeal with prunes to correct constipation.

As symptoms go, a parasite invasion of any kind will cause erratic bowel movements unless your blood type is O. This blood type person has less problems with constipation than most. Eat fruits that hold moisture and indulge in organic figs, mangos, blueberries, oranges, grapes, apples, and pineapples. Blend soaked chia seeds and fresh pineapple with almond or rice milk for a yummy breakfast smoothie. Use stool softeners you can depend on. I have been selling LB-CLN (#14), a product of Nutri-West of Texas, since 1998. It has a perfect mixture of herbs that nudges the colon to purge gently, and you can depend on this product.

Look for gentle laxatives, especially when treating toddlers. Offer them one tablespoon of Grandma's Molasses (blackstrap) in dairy-free milk. If need be, give the child a coffee and chamomile enema. Boil one bag of chamomile tea, steep, and cool. Then add the tea to one cup of black coffee and two cups warm, distilled water. Let the mixture cool and use in an enema bag or fleet enema. Give the child a daily enema for one week or until blockage has been corrected. It is not unusual for the parasites to form a nest among fecal matter hidden somewhere within the approximately sixty feet of the small intestine and colon.

Remember that parasites have no age limit as to whom their hosts may be. Adults will feel tired and anxious, depressed and helpless when infected by this particular amoeba. If working around dirt or dust, it is best to wear a bandana around the mouth and nose to shield from contamination. Dirt and dust is where pinworms, roundworms, tapeworms, and whipworms survive and lay eggs.

If you have carpets, steam clean them regularly and sprinkle baking soda on fabric and then vacuum. Pets must be wormed every three months. If your puppy is dragging his behind on the floor, be forewarned: the dog has worms and is probably infecting you and your children.

Keep vinegar water or Seventh Generation disinfectant handy when traveling or sleeping in unfamiliar accommodations. Many clients have returned from a lovely vacation only to feel sick and run-down rather than refreshed. Frequented hotel rooms are an easy hideout for parasite eggs. If you are traveling and plan on sleeping in an unfamiliar bed, carry a mattress cover and slip it on top of the bottom sheet for protection.

It is sometimes necessary to use a bit of B_{12} to enhance blood production. Use Animal Parade vitamins with iron for children. You may already be praying it forward for sick and unhealthy people. If so, you are in the zone and know how this miracle works. Stick to your morning list of praying it forward and add a healing prayer for the children of God.

Vision Blessing: Christ's White Light

All of my cells are filled with love and light.

— Robyn Nola, Goodreads

In your mind's eye, form a ball of bright white light in your hands. Release the ball from your hands and see it move up and over the top of your head. The white light is spiritually blessed by God's angels. Imagine that this light has energetic healing powers sanctified by God's unconditional love. The white light will clear your mind of all unhealthy thoughts and worries. Imagine the light circling counterclockwise around the top of your head to the bottom of your feet.

Begin to breathe deeply and count ten complete circles, visualizing the ball of light spiraling downward around each chakra (crown, brow, throat, heart, solar plexus, sacral), out the base of your spine, and down the soles of your right foot. Repeat the process in reverse to solidify light in each cell of your body. Feel the instant healing effects as you circle in and around your body's hemisphere. The counterclockwise circular movement of light has a healing effect, and when repeated clockwise, it will seal in God's healing light.

hand holding a ball of light

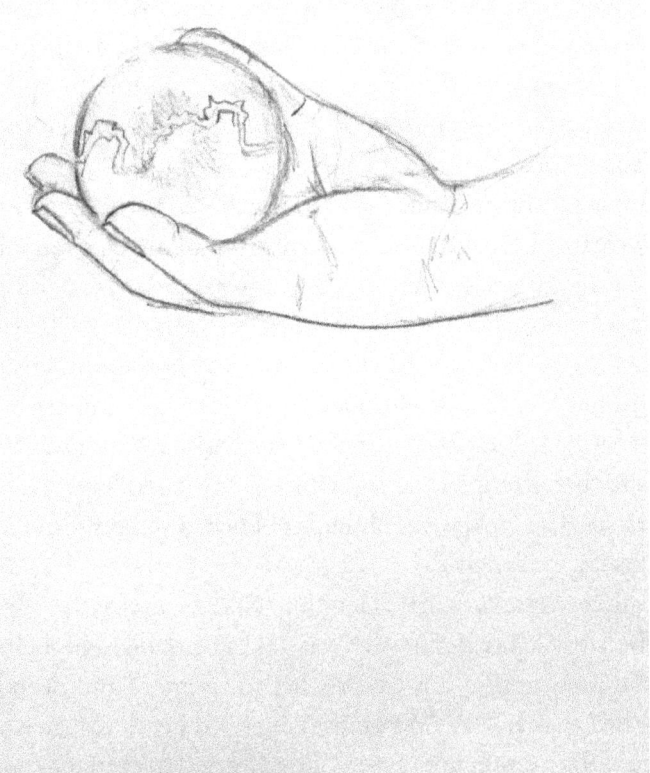

THYROID: TAMPIKA IS BETTER

Tampika came to me with thyroid problems. She told me in her younger days she had been a very popular cheerleader in high school. I was gazing at her sweet face as she continued talking about her problems, but something did not seem quite right to my mind's eye. I kept seeing what I thought to be a ribbon around Tampika's neck. It seemed strange even to me; I had not noticed it when she walked into the clinic.

I was squinting somewhat and continued turning my head until I saw clearly a light blue ribbon with the name of a school written across it in glitter. Just as I was about to excuse myself and go to the ladies' room to splash water on my face, she blurted out words that echoed in the distance. I felt like I was in another dimension when I heard her say, "I was nominated as homecoming queen my senior year." *Okay,* I thought, *I guess I'll soon find out if she was elected.* She told me that after graduating with a 4.0 from college, she became a successful disc jockey, which required her to sit and spin records for long hours every day.

She came to Futuristic Health to find an alternative supplement for the thyroid medicine she was taking because she believed the thyroid prescription was causing her to eat more and sleep less. She confessed to major mood swings that ended her marriage when years of counseling could not save it. She admitted to extreme food binges that eventually caused her to pack on pounds until she tipped the scale at 280. Tampika also confided in me a habit of drinking coffee all day and night while keeping late hours to maintain her career.

When her health became critical, Tampika weighed over three hundred pounds, and she told me she was becoming increasingly irritated by insignificant things. She said once she wanted to die because she left her face powder in the wrong bathroom and had to wait until her sister was finished showering to go and find it. She also told me that all medical doctors she visited were prescribing stronger and stronger antidepressants to regulate her mood swings until she was ultimately diagnosed with schizophrenia. I consider a thyroid problem the number one cause of schizophrenia.

I had to admire Tampika for seeking alternative methods to regulate her weight and stabilize her thyroid. She did not want her life to be controlled by mind-altering drugs. I stepped over to the light switch and dimmed it as I instructed Tampika to lie down and think of the day the school principal announced the winner of homecoming queen her senior year. I put my hand on her throat directly over her thyroid area, knowing it held trapped emotions. Anyone who has read Louise Hay's book *Heal Your Body A–Z: The Mental Causes for Physical Illness and the Way to Overcome Them* may remember her advice.

After I read this book, I learned that the emotion of humiliation is a precursor to thyroid problems. I had Tampika repeat the beautiful affirmation Louise so bravely wrote: "I move beyond old expectations and now allow myself to express freely and creatively." I use this mantra frequently for clients with thyroid problems. Undetected or disclosed, there is always an emotional attachment to all illness. There was a good chance that Tampika's thyroid problems stemmed from a stifling desire to win that position of homecoming queen. I took her quivering hand and noticed tears in her eyes. I held on to them tightly as an offering of warmth and understanding. I asked her to visualize the homecoming banner around her neck as I explained to her that she was a winner.

She had grown to be a very successful adult who had climbed the ladder to executive status and hit the charts as a cool top-ten disc jockey. I told her how spirit had shown me a physic banner displayed around her neck. I let her know it was my gift from God that allowed me to recognize blocks impeding her health. I encouraged her to take a breath and allow the banner to disappear. It was okay that she did not win the position. It would be just fine to go on in life with the thought of allowing someone else to hold the title of homecoming queen. She gushed as she explained to me she had silently held the loss as a crucial failure in her life. We both decided it would be best to let go and let God. I smiled and said, "God has been good to you in many ways. What does it matter now?" That day in my office she released the wounded girl from high school and begin healing her thyroid disease.

Through the use of betaine hydrochloride, an enzymatic supplement to aid in digestion, and a ketogenic diet, her body changed. She has conquered sinking spells, blurry vision, sugar cravings, and carb binges. The shaking and twitching of her eyes and hands has completely stopped. Her hair has thickened and is no longer falling out. Tampika lost one hundred twenty pounds. Today she no longer battles low self-esteem, self-hate, anger issues, and reoccurring paranoia.

When Tampika ate clean foods, her liver and her thyroid would happily assist in food assimilation and hormone support. Eating toxic foods can cause undigested food to stagnate in the stomach, which allows bacteria to travel from the stomach through the windpipe and into the thyroid gland. This cycle of undigested food slows down the thyroid, and the thyroid slows down the digestive system, and undigested food causes depression and lethargy.

Can you imagine the support a clean liver and gallbladder can offer as maintenance to the thyroid gland? Absolutely nothing can correct a thyroid problem as thoroughly as a liver cleanse. I believe the liver and thyroid are first cousins and should work together in harmony. Keep the thyroid gland running like a Maserati by cleaning and purging the liver once a year.

Additives in processed foods can pound a thyroid gland into the ground. Processed dairy, including homogenized milk, has sodium caseinates that inhibit the liver from producing bile for digestion. I believe that if a person ate less fried foods, dairy, and processed animal protein, he or she could effortlessly activate enzymes for digestion.

> Health requires a practice of devotion. It takes
> months and years of rehearsal to master it.
>
> — Sherry Dell

Praying It Forward:

> Finally, brothers and sisters, rejoice! Strive for full restoration,
> encourage one another, be of one mind, live in peace.
> And the God of love and peace will be with you.
>
> — 2 Corinthians 13:11 (NIV)

These words chosen in Praying It Forward were channeled from my spirit in a meditative state to bring forth healing for you. Feel free to alter them as only the Creator knows your needs. As long as you are coming from love and willing to give and receive healing, you are praying it forward.

"Thank you, Creator of life. I am grateful for the sun and the moon allowing my circadian rhythms to reestablish my sleeping and waking schedule. I am blessed to have a perfect thyroid today. I acknowledge that any weight I gained in the past is melting from me today. I believe I am losing weight today, and I am adhering to a healthier diet. Angels, bless me and give me victory over the battle of depression. Fill my heart and mind with thoughts of wisdom and kindness. I choose health and happiness and prioritize it throughout the day. I am instructing my brain to relax and believe that life has good things in store for me. I have excellent sleep at night and possess tremendous energy throughout the day. I support myself with loving words of encouragement. Blessings are discovered in subtle ways as my body fulfills a promise of health and happiness. I am healed, praise God, I am healed."

Golden Rules for Thyroid

You alone decide whether to reach a dead end or live a healthy lifestyle for a long healthy, happy active life.

— Paul C. Bragg

Herbs and vitamins are not meant to replace any medicine prescribed by your healthcare provider. Be sure to follow relevant directions on product labels and consult your pharmacist or physician before using herbs and natural supplements.

Tampika begins her morning by writing a list of nine golden blessings of good things that have come her way. She ends her days by speaking of all the wonderful things that she is grateful for.

Tampika learned to maintain a stable thyroid by steering clear from foods that had preservatives and sodium caseinates. She stopped eating sub sandwiches with lunch meat containing preservatives. She purchased an air fryer to replace a greasy skillet to cook the meaty protein she needed for the ketogenic diet she chose to follow. Tampika also controlled her mood swings by taking valerian root and passion flower. She boosted her metabolism with liquid kelp drops and aided her digestion with betaine hydrochloride. Best of all, Tampika became happy and maintained pride for all the accomplishments she has achieved. She thinks of herself as winner who cherishes the banner of success.

Bladderwrack (*Fucus vesiculosus*) is a natural iodine stimulant for the thyroid that also helps with weight loss. Liquid kelp is a form of thyroid support. Use only a few drops in drinking water daily. Fenugreek is an alkaline herb that suppresses the appetite.

Combine fenugreek with passion flower, horseradish, and milk thistle for liver and thyroid support. Use this combo sparingly yet consistently. Selenium is an essential mineral to support the endocrine glands. Keep walnuts handy for between meal snacking as they are a great source of selenium and you can't beat them for brain power.

Bitter melon is my go-to herb and one of the most popular vegetables grown in Southeast Asia. I have discovered that it has a cleansing effect on all organs, though it is best known for lowering blood sugar. I use it as a mild thyroid stimulant that cleans the pancreas and keeps me from craving sugar. Steer clear from cruciferous vegetables because they can interfere with thyroid function and will crash your energy after eating them. You can slowly begin to eat these brain-shaped vegetables once the thyroid is completely healed.

Clean the thyroid gland with oil swishing. Swish the mouth with organic coconut oil for twenty-one days in the mornings before you brush your teeth. Use one teaspoon oil for swishing and swish continuously for about ten minutes. When you're finished, spit the oil into the trash and rinse your mouth with cool water before brushing your teeth. Use the swishing treatment for twenty-one days on and five days off. Do not swallow any leftover oil. Your thyroid should be clean after two consistent months of oil swishing.

I was raised on crunchy peanut butter sandwiches. Neither I nor my parents knew that I had a peanut allergy. After years of consuming peanut oils, my thyroid had absorbed loads of toxins and began forming small growths inside of the gland. I was a hyperactive wild child, and when I wasn't running and playing, I was in bed sick with sore throats and high fever. After I became a health practitioner, I learned how to clean my thyroid gland by swishing organic coconut oil and taking herbs and vitamins. Though I only have one half of my thyroid left after surgery, I thank God and my thyroid every day for fantastic energy and awesome health.

Use choline, beet powder, and dandelion to support the liver. I love using the mineral Phosfood Liquid—phosphorus is the second most important mineral in the body, and it keeps liver stones, gallstones, and kidney stones in a soluble state. It also supports calcium absorption.

Resist eating sweets and carbohydrates for energy. It is best to eat only natural sweets after a meal so your body will not become dependent on the quick energy sugar provides. Talk yourself into having cherries or green grapes with rice crackers for snacks. Learn to satisfy a sweet tooth the natural way and experience how much smoother your energy is throughout the day. Let the roller-coaster ride end the nutritional way.

Your thyroid is a clock that must be regulated with nutritious food and healthy thoughts. Strive for higher vibrational thoughts and use love as your common denominator to connect with an abundance of healing for yourself and other people.

Chocolate has caffeine in it and is not a healthy choice as it stimulates the thyroid by speeding it up. If you have coffee or hot cocoa, it should be sweetened with coconut oil or stevia and consumed between the hours of six and nine in the morning. Your thyroid is a regulator of energy and controls the pulse of your heart. Get into the groove of supplementing the thyroid with herbs and cleanse this master clock.

Exercise even if you are feeling sluggish because it helps clean toxic wastes from the blood, and believe it or not, you will feel more energetic in time.

Vision Blessing: The Grandfather Clock

I move beyond old limitations and now allow
myself to express freely and creatively.

— Louise Hay

Lie down on the bed and gently close your eyes. With the inhale and exhale of ten deep breaths, visualize a large golden grandfather clock. The clock is a symbol of your body's internal rhythm. As the pendulum swings back and forth, controlling all parts of the clock, mentally connect to this synchronicity. Focus several minutes on the pendulum as it gently sways, keeping perfect time. Hear the steady, consistent ticking and begin to tell your thyroid that it is regulating your body's metabolism just like the pendulum is keeping perfect rhythm for the grandfather clock. Your thyroid is now running as smoothly as the clock. Rest assured that your moods are also stabilizing with each breath you take. Thank the clock for assisting you with this endeavor and open your eyes to a more stable, mindful you. Visit the clock often in your meditations to help your internal clock keep perfect time.

Grandfather clock

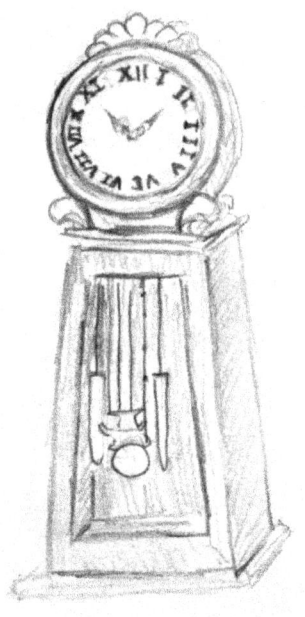

KIDNEYS: NEGATIVE NANCY

Nancy was an exceptional lady who had great faith in God. She told me that she began to lean on God's perfect love after she noticed a pattern in herself of becoming angry with people when things did not go her way. She said it was only by the grace of God that she was able to let go and forgive those whom she believed had initiated the anger. She came into my office with hopes of revealing the mystery behind her problems with persistent kidney infections.

Nancy was raised on a farm and taught to work hard at quite a young age. Her chore as a youngster was collecting fresh eggs from the chicken coop. One bright sunny morning, a mean rooster jumped on top of little Nancy's head and started pecking and scratching at her. Nancy told me that she fainted and couldn't remember what happened after the rooster flogged her. Sadly, her siblings continued to laugh and tease about the rooster for many years. She told me that she was still carrying a pessimistic chip on her shoulders from that fearful day.

Nancy grew up during the Depression when, survival was hard. I sympathized with her and understood life must have been difficult during those unsettled days. She laughed and told me when she graduated from high school, she worked as a carhop. I shrugged my shoulders as if to express, "What the heck is that?" Very quickly, she told me she wore shorts and roller skated around to wait on couples at a drive-in restaurant called Blue Suede Shoes. She skated about serving trays of fries and burgers and resented having to work while she scrapped for loose change in tips to pay for her college.

I told Nancy that I could see a fiery orange glow throughout her waist area right above her low rise blue jeans. She looked ashamed as she confessed that she was even angry with herself for seeking help from a professional like me. "I didn't want to have to pay someone else to help me. I have a burning in my insides, and it hurts for me to urinate." She didn't like confessing her problems to anyone. "I understand," I said. "Sometimes the world is just too heavy to carry all by yourself. Drop the heaviness and confess the ugliness." The words just flew from my mouth. I hoped I had not upset her because by her own confession, she was a walking time bomb.

I discovered that at the very heart of Nancy's problem was an inability to forgive her father for drinking and gambling her family's hard-earned money. She harbored strong emotions that pushed her body into a defensive mechanism known as fight or flight. Emotions of tension and hostility create acidic fluids within the body that can actually interrupt homeostasis—the body's ability to maintain a healthy internal state.

Nancy had been battling kidney infections since she was a little girl. She was still very upset about many things that she believed had gone awry in her life. I hoped she could use a vision blessing to clear old thought patterns of anger and hostility that would change her subconscious beliefs. I explained to her that the kidney's job is to filter impurities from the blood and maintain a perfect level of electrolytes and fluids so our bodies can stay hydrated. Blood passes into the kidneys to remove waste and excess salt as well as other fluids that may not be thoroughly eliminated.

When kidneys become weak and sluggish, uric acid tips the pH balance to the acidic side. Kidney infections become more dominating and can contaminate and infect the bladder, ureters, and urethra. Uric acid spills into the bloodstream and weakens the heart muscles. Imagine a poison liquid filtering into small streams and rivers that leads to a large pool of water. This is what happens when uric acid seeps into the blood veins and arteries and makes its way to the large pool of blood pumping from your heart muscle. Kidney stones are responsible for hernias in the stomach and the groin.

Kidney and bladder stones are likely to cause back pain and hip joint deterioration. This is why I say, "Out with dairy and sodas." Other symptoms of kidney stones are shooting pains that run up, down, and behind the legs, knees, and low back. Kidney stones can eventually cause serious hip problems that may require replacement surgery. Weak kidneys impede hearing too because the kidneys rule the eyes and ears in Chinese meridian theory. Anytime a person has a hard time hearing me, I try to respond with loving words and repeat myself a little louder; I know the person having hearing problems has had his or her share of anger and misery. Another symptom that may physically manifest in your body when dealing with kidney problems is swelling around the knees and ankles to the point of arthritic pain.

Obviously, you see how important it is to give your kidneys much love and appreciation. Water your kidneys like you would a hibiscus plant and use fruit juices and electrolytes as fertilizers to keep them filtering. Love is the key word when you are experiencing kidney problems. Take these words into strong consideration, or you will be battling two kidneys that have become cantankerous giants. Calm your mind with peaceful thoughts, and your kidneys will stay calm for you.

Ms. Nancy decided to write down on paper her blessing every day and count the goodness that God was bringing into her life. She uses her vision blessing to ensure that her life is sweet and easy. Through the use of betaine hydrochloride, an enzymatic supplement to aid in digestion, and a vegetarian diet, she is managing her bladder infections.

She has conquered blurry vision, hearing loss, joint pain, and the persistent urgency to urinate. She has been able to control her anger, and she no longer gets upset at the drop of a hat. She drinks parsley and green tea for a morning clean sweep drink.

If you suspect kidney stones are trapped in your body, try using the herb hydrangea. Take three capsules each day with water. Use stone breaker in water and take calsol. Sprinkle some asparagus powder into warm water, let this mixture set for fifteen minutes and drink each night before bed.

Feed these gentle giants clear liquids, fruits, and vegetables and then abracadabra, the kidneys will be your servants for many years.

Praying It Forward

Let all bitterness, and wrath, and anger, and clamor, and evil speaking, be put away from you, with all malice: And be ye kind to one another, even as God for Christ's sake hath forgiven you.

— Ephesians 4:31–32 (KJV)

These words chosen in Praying It Forward were channeled from my spirit in a meditative state to bring forth healing for you. Feel free to alter them as only the Creator knows your needs. As long as you are coming from love and willing to give and receive, you are praying it forward.

Thank you for this new day. It is a beautiful day and may be the only day that I have left on this marvelous planet. I am blessed to have friends who have listened to my problems. I am a good listener and speak less and less about negative events that are going on in my world today. Thank you for helping me to receive healing through speaking positive words. I am very blessed and happy to know goodness when I see, feel, and hear it. Bless those people who cannot hear and those who walk in pain. My kidneys are healed, thank you. Thank you for turning my ears inward and allowing me to hear my words and speak only kindness. Thank you for courage to turn away from stressful thoughts today. Thank you for the awesome healing powers in organic foods. Thank you for guided visualization and meditation. Thank you for giving the planet clean water to drink. Clean water comes to our homes, countries, and the world we live in.

Golden Rules for Kidneys

Life isn't happening to you; life is responding to you.

— Rhonda Byrne, *The Power*

Herbs and vitamins are not meant to replace any medicine prescribed by your healthcare provider. Be sure to follow relevant directions on product labels and consult your pharmacist or physician before using herbs and natural supplements.

Kidney Activator by Nature's Sunshine is an excellent source for cleaning kidneys. Drink extra water with any herbal remedies. Boil three cups of water and throw a handful of cleaned parsley into the pot as you take it off the hot burner. Put the lid on the pot to steep tea for five minutes and drink it warm. Parsley tea will balance electrolytes and clean the kidneys.

If low back pain is prevalent, it is a possible sign of kidney stones. Discontinue eating dairy and use rice or almond milk in place of cow's milk. Take three hydrangea capsules per day to ease kidney stones from the body. Eat asparagus or buy powdered asparagus and drink one-fourth teaspoon in warm water every night for two weeks. Let the asparagus powder dissolve for fifteen minutes before drinking it.

Purchase Stone Breaker from the company Herb Pharm to dissolve persistent stones. Use as directed on the bottle but start out in low doses to be sure your body is healing properly. Standard Process sells Phosfood Liquid, and this product is definitely worth the small investment. Use Stone Breaker or Phosfood Liquid in water or apple juice.

Drink organic apple juice and eat organic apple sauce to soften any kidney stones. Use ground flaxseed mixed with a bit of cottage cheese to slow down the absorption. Take black currant seed oil if you are experiencing hearing loss. You must confess to yourself a pattern of negative thinking before you can hear your words clearly. Let go and let God help your kidneys to heal.

Drink weak lemon water at lunch or indulge in mild green tea throughout the day. The support that green tea gives to the kidneys is amazing. Try substituting coffee with roasted dandelion tea, though I know for us coffee fiends that is a tall order.

Be sure to use only sweeteners that are natural and organic sugars of good quality. Use stevia as a sweetener by the company Sweet Leaf. Be careful with stevia that has erythritol included as a blend. Erythritol is a fermented corn sugar that can also be used as an insecticide. There are tons of artificial sugars that claim to be harmless, but the truth is most people have a really rough time digesting artificial sugars, which can remain stagnant in the bloodstream and damage the kidneys and bladder.

If you use artificial sugar, notice if your urination activity has slowed down or become stagnant. Check to see if the color of your urine is clear with perhaps just a faint bit of yellow. Dark-colored urine and short trips to the toilet are symptoms that your kidneys are not filtering correctly. Low back pain, hip pain, knee pain, or sacral pain are all signs of kidney stones. Drink water, drink water, drink water. Feel love, speak love, stay in love. Resist criticism and speak your kidneys into healing. You were made from love, so continue the chain of healing with a feeling of joy and happiness.

Vision Blessing: The Curtain, the Wind, the Window

When you are happy you can forgive a great deal.

— Diana, Princess of Wales

In your mind's eye, see yourself standing in front of an open window with orange curtains that are blowing in the summer wind. The window is completely open, and you find yourself standing directly in front of it. The curtains blow on either side of the open window. The warm wind has a fragrance of roses wafting from a beautiful flower garden behind this window of healing. This is a safe place to be while you enjoy being alone with your thoughts. Allow your body to absorb the warmth of the sun as you inhale and exhale ten long, deep breaths. Smell the scent of the flowers. Stand still and allow yourself to be healed from negative situations harbored in your past. Be it yesterday or years ago, it is time to release, relax, and let go of the outdated, unwanted pain in your body. Bring the memory of a trauma to the forefront of your mind and let the wind sweep away the trauma. The wind is cleaning and clearing emotions that no longer serve you. Take one step closer to the window and feel the curtain brush by your cheek. Let this be a reminder that you are a living ball of energy that has abundant light to shine for eternity. Forgive anyone who has offended you, and don't forget to include yourself.

Be good to your soul. Make it glad it picked you for the existence of this lifetime.

The Window the wind and the Curtain

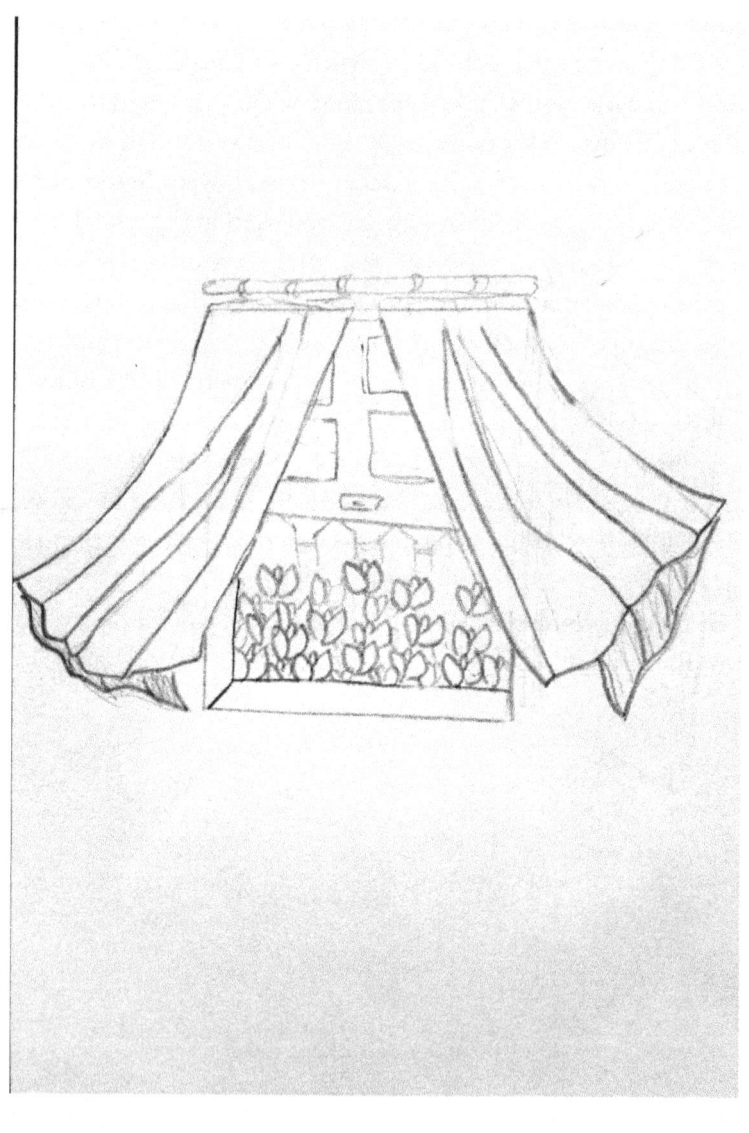

SARAH-JAN SAVES HER GALLBLADDER

I have had the pleasure of helping many clients work through a gallbladder attack, and in the spring of 2015, a classic gallbladder case walked into my office. When Sarah-Jan entered the lobby, she was holding her right side. She explained to me that when playing tennis, she suddenly doubled over in pain. I asked her to lie down so I could gently examine a gallbladder acupressure point on the right side of her body directly below the breast. She squinted when I touched it as if it hurt and told me that she felt sick to her stomach and was experiencing pain on the right and left sides of her neck and shoulders. I tested her acupressure points in the area of her gallbladder and bile ducts to determine that she was in full-blown attack mode.

I asked her what she had eaten in the last twenty-four hours. She excitedly told me she had baked cheese enchiladas for her family the night before her big tennis match. It is important to backtrack the food that is responsible for the gallbladder attack. Discovering which food has pushed the person over the edge into a painful fit of indigestion is the first note to self so that it doesn't happen again. In most cases, spicy foods like BBQ or hot chicken wings will be a precursor to a gallbladder attack that sometimes feels like a heart attack. Long before an attack, the person has consumed more than his or her share of trans fats and processed food.

I have learned from experience that once a person has gallbladder problems, cleansing and flushing gallstones must be a ritual undertaken every year or so to keep the organ healthy. Seventy-five percent of the food we eat should be harvested from the ground and not contain GMOs, fertilizers, and preservatives. If this is not taken into consideration, there will be reoccurring problems.

Sarah-Jan shared with me that a few of her friends had opted to have their gallbladders removed once they experienced an attack. After surgery, her friends were still going through bouts of diarrhea, headaches, back pain, and of course indigestion. Sarah-Jan felt she needed to go to the emergency room and seek medical help but was afraid the doctors would suggest a cholecystectomy. Sarah-Jan told me she intended on keeping all of her organs, and I agree with her sportsmanship attitude of "winner take all." Had I caved in to a hysterectomy at age thirty-three, my precious Milan would not be here today.

I take pride in the overwhelming number of gallbladders I have helped to save and for the many clients who are as determined as Sarah-Jan. There was one thing that Sarah-Jan and I had in common, and this was a spiritual belief that negative thoughts could cause problems within the body—thoughts of insecurities and worry can throw a monkey wrench into a healthy lifestyle. Sarah-Jan and I both knew that her thinking was clouded in the days before her attack. She was anxious about the tennis match and secretly was concerned about whether she could win the match.

Suddenly I had a serious twinge of fear travel into my throat and felt as if I were drowning and needed to swim up to the top of the ceiling. "What in the heck has been going on, Sarah-Jan?" I asked. I was obviously feeling her emotions of overwhelming fear. It is not unusual for me to meet a person at my office late at night or early in the mornings if they are experiencing a gallbladder attack. Many times, a gallbladder attack will feel like a tight, squeezing pressure in the chest and mimic a heart attack. According to the look in Sarah-Jan's face and her body language, she was hurting big time.

Clients having a gallbladder attack will feel clammy, nauseous, and sometimes they will feel as if the air is being knocked from their bodies. I held on to my rib cage and knew that I was feeling her pain. I didn't question it because many times I use my intuitive gift to understand more thoroughly what a patient is experiencing physically, emotionally, and mentally.

I had no choice but to accept this stifling energy that was engulfing me from head to toe. Sarah-Jan held her head and complained of a headache and neck pain that was cramping the right side of her neck and shoulder. She used her thumb to scroll up her back and pointed to the hot spot of pain. I can honestly say that unless a person is eating clean, and by that I mean eliminating dairy, processed meats, and all chemically processed foods, they can find themselves in the emergency room facing a cholecystectomy.

The gallbladder is a little bitty hollow gland that weighs about one half an ounce and stores the powerful enzyme bile. I have stressed how important bile is for proper digestion of fats, oils, and protein. I believe that without the aid of the gallbladder, meat is sparsely digested. After days, months, and even years of accumulated bacteria, thick bile hardens in ducts and around the organ, causing stones.

When preparing for the cleanse, take extra enzymes. There are no cement walls in our bodies designed to keep bacterial gasses from seeping into our mouths, where bacteria can cause pressure in the frontal lobe of the brain. Depression and mental anxiety is more than likely a symptom of gallstones. Bacteria from undigested food in the stomach is responsible for mouth and gum disease. The gallbladder is a very delicate and integral part of the hepatic loop. This loop consists of the four-pound liver that houses and protects the tiny gallbladder. The left and right hepatic ducts connect to the cystic duct, forming one common duct that is critical to the delivery of bile and mandatory for complete digestion. The common bile duct stems into and through the pancreas, where it empties bile into the stomach for the digestion of fats, oils, and protein.

When a person craves excess sugar and carbs, I see it as a red flag indicating that the client is depleted of bile as a crucial enzyme. Pancreatic enzymes are pushing to work harder for the digestion of protein in the small intestine. Ducts are tiny roadways that deliver precious enzymes and other fluids into the organs. The right and left hepatic duct run side by side into the cystic duct that merges into the common bile duct. It is this singular duct, the common bile duct, that stretches completely through the pancreas delivering bile for the digesting of protein, fats, and oil. In other words, Mr. Bile Duct and Mrs. Pancreatic Duct are man and wife. They are willing to work as a team as long as there is compromise.

Post a sticky note to your refrigerator that reads, "A clean bile duct equals good cholesterol, mental clarity, a great sex drive, and a diabetes-free life."

A dirty liver and gallbladder clogs the internal wheel, confusing the digestive system. When this happens, bowel movements become sporadic, causing migraine headaches and energy to go down the toilet instead.

Sarah-Jan made three visits to my office the week of her gallbladder fiasco and was very compliant. She ate organic apple sauce, drank the organic juice, and followed the directions on the gallbladder flush. She had to flush her gallbladder three times in three months. Back-to-back cleanses are not often recommended, but I insist on repeating this process if the gallbladder is slow to revive.

It is sometimes necessary to take coffee enemas for two weeks during the gallbladder cleanse. The minute the coffee hits the rectum, it opens the liver and bile ducts; this procedure allows the stones to purge all toxins.

My clients are amazed at the collection of stones they cleanse from their bodies during the gallbladder flush; they honestly believe they are doing me a favor by displaying them on my office desk in clear plastic baggies. Personally, I am not fond of the collections of stones, but it is always nice to have proof that the stones have been thoroughly removed. Sarah-Jan continues to play tennis and eats a strict vegan diet. If I see her name appear on my cell phone, I have a pretty good idea that she's fallen off the wagon and her gallbladder and liver are giving her heck. Guess she couldn't say no cheese on the enchiladas. The fact is, once a gallbladder has misbehaved, it must be on probation for life.

> Good health is a simple choice of living to eat the foods
> we love or learning to eat the foods that love us back.

— Sherry Dell

Praying It Forward

> And we have known and believed the love that
> God has for us. God is love, and he who abides
> in love abides in God, and God in him.

— 1 John 4:16 (NIV)

These words chosen in Praying It Forward were channeled from my spirit in a meditative state to bring forth healing for you. Feel free to alter them as only the Creator knows your needs. As long as you are coming from love and willing to give and receive, you are praying it forward.

I am healed with organic foods; I am healed with clear water. Food, water, and clean thoughts are healing me. I feed my body clean foods. Clean living is the easiest choice I have ever made. I effortlessly make the best choices possible when it comes to healing my body. Natural foods and clean water are my first priority when my health is concerned. I absolve myself from caffeinated drinks. I love drinking tea and water. I am good to my gallbladder and it is good to me.

There are many times when we simply need to connect to love. I can tell if my love frequencies are not in sync by the way I feel. These are the times when I gently sing a song of praise. Music is helpful, and even if you can only hum, you will discover that in a matter of minutes you will begin to feel uplifted. Singing and humming will bring a sedative of peace to your heart and soul. When you sing words of blessings, you are spreading love and blessing to yourself. Your sound frequencies will lift the vibrations of the planet. I simply sing a song of healing by using the tune to "Mary Had a Little Lamb." Blessings, blessings, I am healed; blessings, blessings, I am healed. Blessings, blessings, I am healed; I am healed today.

God, I pray today blessings for someone who feels he or she is not worthy to receive healing. I remove fear, anger, and unhealthy thoughts from my mind. I know that my organs are healing. It is easy to choose nutritious foods that supply my temple of God. My heart and my body are clean. I am healed from sickness, and I have the power to speak health into existence. I have the desire to gravitate toward nourishing foods for healing. I receive many blessings of health.

Golden Rules

When I stand before God at the end of my life I would
hope that I would have not a single bit of talent left
and could say, I used everything you gave me.

— Erma Bombeck

Herbs and vitamins described in each chapter are not meant to replace any medicine prescribed by your healthcare provider. Be sure to follow relevant directions on product labels and consult your pharmacist or physician before using herbs and natural supplements.

It is vital to keep bile ducts clean in order for the digestive system to work. Drink apple juice daily or eat applesauce or take apple pectin. Beets are a powerful healing agent to the gallbladder; they have a thinning effect on bile as it enters the stomach. Cut back on fast foods and fried meat. Look for trans fat on packaged snacks as a first or second ingredient. These oils, when eaten over a period of time, will put the hurt on your gallbladder.

Sometimes a gallstone will travel from the liver or gallbladder and become lodged in one of the three bile ducts. This is when to take my trusty go-to vitamin choline bitartrate. If any supplement can heal the planet, it is choline. Choline has a Roto-Rooter effect and softens calcified stones that are trapped inside of the bile ducts. This vitamin will certainly clear the pathway for your liver to release bile.

Go organic and avoid products that say GMO or MSG as these chemicals are additives that clog up the delicate gallbladder. Eat steel-cut oats four mornings a week and have organic eggs the other three. Organic vegetables seasoned with organic lemon or lime juice will help you to digest more easily.

Coconut oil and ghee are awesome butter replacements and taste delicious too. When my clients eliminate processed dairy such as yellow cheese and milk, they stop having gallbladder problems. If you are vegan, you can reach for butter substitutes that do not have soy in them. In my opinion, you can't go wrong with Kerrygold butter when searching for a pure form of cow's butter. This butter is made from grass-fed cattle in Ireland, where the pastures have not had chemicals sprayed on them. Use sparingly and slow down on processed breads and pastas. I should not have to mention sodas, but for your sake, I will remind you that these poisons really dry out the gallbladder. Stopping this one terribly bad habit will save you thousands of dollars from trips to the emergency room.

Symptoms of an unhealthy gallbladder are pimple breakouts on the face, neck, back, and arms. Some gallbladder sufferers also complain of feeling sick in the morning and sometimes throwing up when trying to have a bowel movement. Constipation followed by diarrhea are usually symptoms of a weak gallbladder. Headaches are very common when having gallbladder problems. This problem can also cause short term memory loss that may develop into Alzheimer's or Parkinson's disease.

Omit this fear from your future by feeding the gallbladder unprocessed food. Other symptoms of poor bile production from a sick gallbladder are depression, anxiety, stiff neck, aching shoulders, and pain in mid back. Don't forget that the thyroid gland and gallbladder are close cousins. If the gallbladder is unhealthy, it will cause symptoms of a sluggish thyroid. For those of you who have had your gallbladder removed, use the same protocol and take extra enzymes. If you are still having diarrhea, there is a possibility that there is a gallstone trapped inside of the common bile duct. Use a teaspoon of arrowroot powder mixed in water to aid with indigestion and eat a scrapped apple to calm down diarrhea. The cleansing will take time to complete, but if you stick with apple pectin, beets, choline, and Phosfood Liquid, you will see results.

Make vegetables your mainstay and have organic chicken or wild-caught fish once or twice a week only when you feel a craving for protein. Stay positive and reach for healthy foods. Rice is a natural stimulator for the digestive system and acts as a sponge for toxins and acids. Cook with oils that can handle a high smoke point.

Most refined oils have a higher smoke point than the less refined variety. Refined oils are impossible to digest, and I believe this is what gets us into gallbladder trouble. You can make use of organic avocado oil when frying foods using temperatures up to 500 degrees. Avocado oil helps break down cholesterol and is great for frying. Use cold-pressed oils such as extra virgin olive oil for salads and dressings and low temperature stir fry. Stay clear from peanut oil, soybean oil, corn oil, and other refined vegetable oils.

Never underestimate your body's ability to heal.

— Sherry Dell

Vision Blessing: Walking Down Easy Street

Close your eyes and imagine you are walking down a street that is deep and wide. Take a mental picture of the street sign that reads "Easy Street" etched in green and gold. Store this image in your memory as a reminder that this street is the healing path you enjoy walking on.

Begin taking deep breaths as you slide into deeper relaxation and begin repeating the words "easy street."

"Easy street" symbolizes a quick and easy reminder to stay focused on your path to health. Your health is improving by using positive words of self-prophecy. All you need do is see the street name appear in your mind's eye. Once you cross this street in your vision blessing, it will automatically help you to make better food choices for the entire day. Say the words "easy street" right before you go to sleep, and you will wake up on the road to health. Let health travel into your home, down the sidewalk, and into the streets to spread healing throughout your community.

Street Sign that reads Easy street

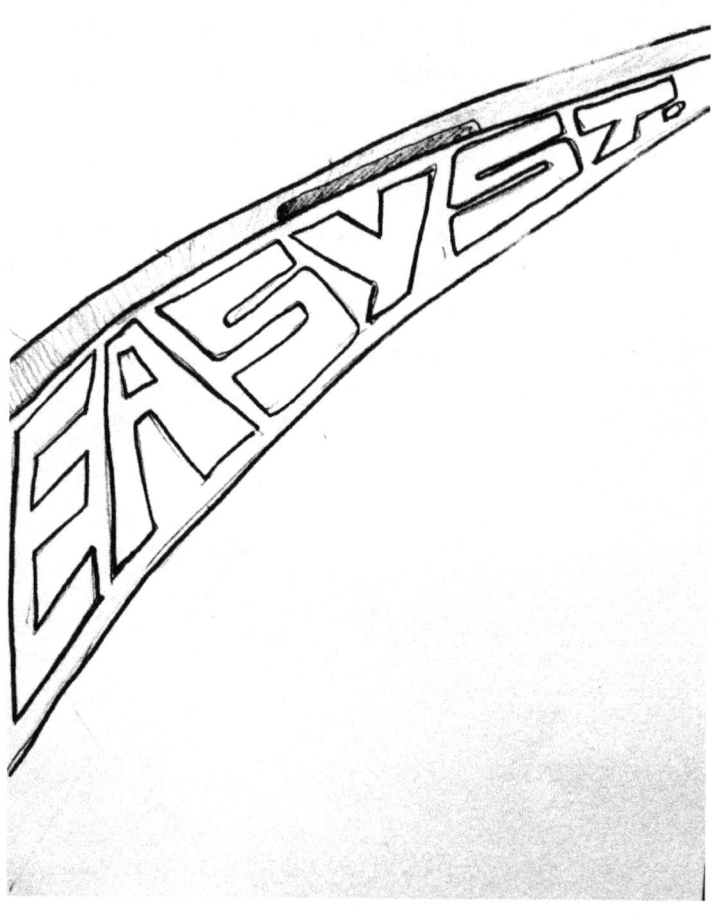

PROSTATE CANCER: MR. FITNESS

I braced Hank for the fact that parasite infections predispose people to cancer. It was 2010, and Futuristic Health was steadily seeing new clients arrive for testing and healing. I recognized a name that appeared on my appointment book and smiled thinking of the small world we live in. This man was a fitness instructor who had raised the bar in defense training.

Hank explained to me he was planning a life of longevity, and because he and I highly respected each other, he felt he could trust my professional opinion to help him with his latest medical report. His PSA level was well over 4.0, and he was all in on finding a way to lower these numbers. PSA stands for prostate-specific antigen and measures malignant as well as normal cells of the prostate gland. Hank wasn't anxious in the least about the medical report, he just wanted to cover all his bases and heal his body as fast as possible.

I hesitated to say the word *parasite* because so many doctors and medical advisers pooh-pooh this hypothesis. But when I looked into his eyes, I could tell that he had done his homework. He agreed with me wholeheartedly and confided in me that this possibility did not surprise him. He had spent time as a guest speaker in various countries around the globe. I do believe that a person can be more susceptible to cuisine contamination in foreign countries because the body has not built up a defense to amoebas in the food and water.

Let's not rule out the possibility of parasite infestations developing through importation and exportation of food in the United States.

As we spoke, I sensed a degree of regret thickening the air in the room. I saw dark circles under his eyes, and I remembered that I had noticed those circles several years before I opened my clinic as a health counselor. I was attending a meeting with a group of business owners the day that I noticed him across the crowded room. I wondered then why he looked so tired.

Quickly, my mind drifted back to my office just in time to hear him speak of his on and off successful business in the physical training industry. I saw before my mind's eye an image of a teeter-totter. I remembered playing on one of them as a small child. I also knew it took two individuals to use this recreational toy. He was catching me up on his past and telling me how his new dojo was run by a partner he had known all of his life. He was hanging his head and grumbling about the good and bad times. "I know it has been hard on you working with a partner who may not see eye to eye with your old-fashioned rules," I said suddenly, then put my hands over my mouth. "Sorry!" I said. He looked at me with a smile as if he was glad I said it. "No," he replied, "I have always been a guy who wanted things ran my way. I am ready for a change. Tell me what to do." *Now that was really easy*, I thought. I gave him a quick nod that told him I was ready to move on and help.

I knew from the vision and the dark circles under his eyes that he had worked hard at gaining success. In my opinion, he needed a major mental shift for the odds to swing in his favor. He was depressed and unhappy with his diagnosis of cancer. Love and forgiveness should now be his first rule of thought. He spoke softly, almost in monotone, "I just want to be healthy now." I responded by saying something I would say to myself when my parents would quarrel: "Just be happy."

The prostate gland is a part of the male reproductive system. It is a walnut-size gland located inside the body between the bladder and urethra. A prostate gland that grows too large can place pressure on the bladder and cause discomfort. Men with an enlarged prostate will excuse themselves several times to urinate during the course of a forty-minute office visit. This urgency is a sign that pressure is building due to trapped toxins in and around the kidneys, bladder, and the prostate gland. I recommend a kidney and bladder cleanses using asparagus and a few drops of edible lemon oil in water.

It didn't take Hank two minutes to straight up ask me what parasite medicine he needed to start taking and which foods he should eliminate to control his PSA numbers. Hank was looking for a silver bullet to squash this potentially life-threatening health problem of prostate cancer, and he was eager to use the vision blessings to speed up his healing. I told him to forget about cheese, dairy, and red meat. He needed to begin juicing organic carrots, celery, and kale. Food goes into the body and must be digested in order to leave the body in a state of health. Bacteria can exit from the body in four ways: urination, bowel movements, breath, and sweat. You must digest the waste going out. Digestive enzymes will keep the stomach juices flowing in order to properly digest. Occasional probiotics like cabbage, yogurt, and cottage cheese help supply the colon with friendly bacteria.

Many of my clients self-educate by studying pioneers from years ago. These naturalists laid down the tracks for organic healing in Europe and America. Some of these pioneers make use of Hulda Clark's formulas and inventions for parasite elimination. Hank was extremely open to avenues of nutritional healing. He had read that all cancer begins with a parasite infection. I was happy that I did not have to convince him to do a parasite cleanse.

One popular therapy I recommend to anyone showing signs of cancer cells is intravenous (IV) chelation therapy. For those of you who are not aware of this process, it involves IV injections of a chelating agent called EDTA (*ethylenediaminetetraacetic acid*), which is a synthetic acid. EDTA binds to heavy metals and minerals in the blood so that they can be excreted in the urine. In my mind, chelation is especially useful when a kidney, bladder, or prostate gland shows signs of swelling.

Anyone who has received news of cancer thriving in his or her body should immediately begin drinking Jason Winters' Tea. The tea consists of red clover, sage, and chaparral; it is an ancient remedy proven to shrink tumors and diminish cancer cells. Asparagus powder is also known to raise the immune system to fight cancer cells. The balm of Gilead is a zinc paste that has many health benefits, including the ability to minimize or eliminate the symptoms of cancer.

Look into natural cancer healing centers that do stem cell and hyperbaric therapy. New Hope Unlimited is a trustworthy clinic in San Luis Potosí, Mexico. Never give on the hope of healing. Look up to God and ask the universe for a miracle. Your body will respond favorably to a positive attitude with an abundance of gratitude. Be thankful for alternative healing and organic foods. If you have cancer of any kind, please eliminate all sugar and red meats and search the farmer's market for organic fish and chicken that do not have hormones. Please don't be fooled when the package says "no hormones added." It is possible the baby chicken has already had a big dose of estrogen. If the product is labeled organic or you have found a co-op as a dependable source for your meat, congratulations!

Any physical fitness instructor will be the first to tell you that exercise is a high-ranking priority to combat illness. Second to exercise is to maintain a joyous attitude and fill your life with laughter and happiness. Your brain emits serotonin and dopamine when you have joy in your heart. Take a few minutes each day to initiate a euphoric state of being and get excited about healing. Laughter, joy, and peace will initiate healing chemistry throughout your body's T cells.

One healing strategy Hank and I agreed on is detoxifying the body and keeping the body clear of added chemicals. For colds, sinus problems, and joint and muscle pain, choose wisely from a natural source of vitamin C. Black elderberry liquid is very high in vitamin C and it targets viruses. Liposomal C can be taken twice a day with food. Turmeric controls inflammation and pain. Use a teaspoon of elderberry, echinacea, or goldenseal to build the immune system. White willow bark and turmeric are great for pain relief and help the liver to eliminate toxic die off. Melatonin fights cancer but should not be taken in high doses. Use the herb mullein as a healing substitute for drying out sinus infections. Drugstore medicines and over-the-counter pain remedies have an extreme drying effect on our precious livers. We need the liver clean to help digest toxins from the body. If the liver is full of chemicals, the kidneys are overworked. Toxic kidneys can be harsh to the bladder, and the bladder will inadvertently poison the prostate. You see, there really are no cement walls separating the organs inside of the human body. All of our organs must communicate with one another in harmony.

Hank embraced the detoxing phase of his healing by cutting out all foods with preservatives, hormones, and sugar. He is still living a cancer-free life. His love of health and fitness helped him combat his illness. Oh yes, and he replaced anxiety with love and forgiveness. He realized that being right was not always the most important thing.

If you are the person in your city, town, or
village who advocates health and fitness, you are
changing the planet one work out at a time.

— Sherry Dell

Praying It Forward:

Then God said, "I give you every sea bearing plant
on the face of the whole earth and every tree that has
fruit with seed in it. They will be yours for food."

— Genesis 1:29 (NIV)

These words chosen in Praying It Forward were channeled from my spirit in a meditative state to bring forth healing for you. Feel free to alter them as only the Creator knows your needs. As long as you are coming from love and willing to receive, you are praying it forward.

"Today I claim total and complete healing. I am confident that my body is responding to the healing herbs and alkalizing food I choose to eat daily. I can feel my prostate gland shrinking as tremendous pressure releases from my stomach and lower extremities. I claim my purpose to live as a strong and healthy man. I especially pray for those who are not treating their bodies as temples of God. I pray today for cancer patients be filled with the Creator's healing light. This light in my life is gathering strength minute by minute, and its enormity continues to heal me from within.

For the Cancer Patient's Mental Healing

I am regaining strength, and I claim my healing each morning when I awaken. I release any hate, anger, or worries that may have entered my thoughts in the past. I forgive myself for any wrong I may have done. Today, I claim victory over illness, and I am not in a hurry to be first in line. I am whole, I am healthy, and I feel surges of energy during the day. I smile and laugh in confidence that my body has shifted into the zone of **healing**. Each morning when I awaken and every evening as I close my eyes, I say the words, "I am healing, I am healed, I have healed. Thank you, God; thank you, prayer-givers, thank you. I am well, I am healthy, and I am in mental and physical alignment to receive God's healing light today."

If you point your finger at someone you know is
abusing his or her health, turn your finger inward
to be sure your body is nourishing your soul.

— Sherry Dell

Golden Rules

Attend not only to how food tastes but to
how it alters your well-being.

— Judith Orloff, MD, author of *Positive Energy*

Herbs and vitamins described in each chapter are not meant to replace any medicine prescribed by your healthcare provider. Be sure to follow relevant directions on product labels and consult your pharmacist or physician before using herbs and natural supplements.

My approach to battling cancer and other viral infections is a familiar pattern of eliminating dairy, sugar, and red meat as well as all processed foods. Substitute your sweet tooth with stevia by SweetLeaf or Swerve. Eat organic vegetables, chicken, and fish to keep up with protein for cell reproduction. Steer clear from foods that contain high carbohydrates. Pick a color and associate it with healing. For instance, if you choose turquoise, each time you see it, remind yourself that you are cancer free. The herbs passion flower, withiania, and Bach flowers steady nerves. Turmeric can be used for pain and calming the nerves and is also excellent for eliminating toxins in the liver. Avoid tomatoes, peppers, and eggplant if you have trouble with aching legs. Check into the possibility of finding pure hemp oil to diminish cancer cells, anxiety, insomnia, and depression.

Artemisia and black walnut will start the parasite elimination process. Use in liquid form if possible and begin with ten drops of each herb in water daily. Use ten drops of liquid cayenne pepper each day and keep the alkaline flowing. Locate Jason Winters' Tea and drink four to six cups daily. Add to water a few drops of grapefruit seed extract—this seed has healing effects on viral infections and is 100 percent alkaline.

Asparagus powder is good for softening stones and cleaning kidneys; it helps to clear out any calcified and hardened bacteria that has been trapped in the bladder and ureters. Eliminate all melon from the diet and stop eating sugar of any kind. Read labels and be aware of how much added sugar is in everything.

Use a mild probiotic to begin your healing regime. If constipation persists, take less probiotic and drink Smooth Move tea. Intestinal Freedom is recommended to keep the bowels regulated. Work a coffee enema into your morning routine. Use one cup cool organic coffee, and remember it is not necessarily for bowel movements but to jumpstart your liver to eliminate bacteria from every cell every day.

For five days at the beginning of each month, drink the juice from half a lemon and 1/8 teaspoon baking soda in one cup water. This old-fashioned remedy helps to alkalize the blood. Viruses live in an acidic environment, and five days will be plenty of time to alkalize your body; this is another case where less is best. Locate liposomal vitamin C and work up to ten thousand milligrams daily. If angina, or heart pain, is a problem when taking vitamin C in high doses, back off to find your body's limit.

Try not to backslide on your diet and vitamin supplements. If you do miss a day and decide to eat barbecue or chicken wings, don't get sidetracked. Pick up where you left off. Begin speaking positive words to your body and direct yourself to get back on the healing track. Too many times my clients will be upset for backsliding only to continue the slump. Get back on schedule, forgive yourself, and move onward and upward.

Drink plenty of water and do not eat high-carbohydrate fruits. Unfortunately, apples are high in carbs and are not the best fruit to fight cancer. Take the herb saw palmetto three times daily. This herb has beneficial effects on shrinking a man's enlarged prostate gland. According to the Mayo Clinic, more than two million American men use saw palmetto to treat an enlarged prostate.

Be sure to advise your medical doctor of any herbs you are taking to naturally combat this or any medical condition. Play it safe and check for contraindication when using herbs for healing.

Eat pumpkin seeds daily to sweep away toxins from the prostate gland. I stir-fry them with asparagus tips. Pumpkin seeds contain free-radical-scavenging antioxidants. They improve testosterone levels, which will help keep the immune system strong for any man who is going through this illness.

"I am healed," are my favorite new words.

— Sherry Dell

Vision Blessing: God's Chemotherapy

From time immemorial, healthy people have held sick people hostage. I believe hostage holding of the sick is immoral, fundamentally unethical, and needs to be stopped.

— Hulda Regehr Clark

The mind is our greatest tool. It can create a new belief system that informs cells to combat illness. The right side of the brain does not recognize the difference between fantasy and reality. Therefore, with vision blessings, we are instructing the immune system to defeat all odds in any circumstance concerning our health. Train your brain to obey and stay focused on a positive outcome.

Sit quietly in a chair and slowly inhale and exhale ten breaths to clear your mind and prepare for a cylinder to begin descending from the top of the ceiling. Visualize this tube emitting electrical frequencies of a purple light that will charge your body with healing energies.

On your last inhale, continue imagining the cylinder is hovering over your entire body, showering God's chemotherapy on you. The electrical energy is purging and cleaning your body deep within its cellular level. During the day, as you go about your business, think about the smell of seaweed and taste the salt from the ocean on your tongue. The sound and taste instantly remind you of this magnificent healing light. Once you have imprinted your sensory memory, you will see in your mind's eye the purple light of God coming to heal you many times throughout the day.

Feel confident that this light is charging your cells with total and complete immune support. Be blessed with the Creator's omnipotent healing. Whenever you ask, this light will bring you waves of healing. All you need to do is think of the tube emitting light, and your right brain will respond to healing on all levels, all day, always. Believe in your innate abilities and cancel any fear or worries. Let this time of healing be 100 percent in your favor.

chair

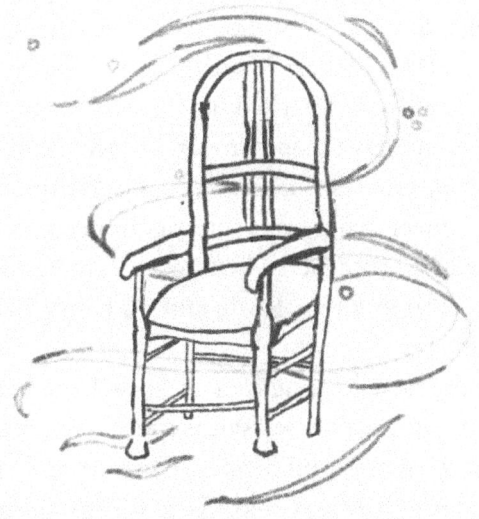

DIGESTION: THE BOY
IN THE BAND

It was a busy day in March when I noticed my cell phone lighting up as I turned my Jeep into my designated parking space at the Futuristic Health office in Fort Worth, Texas. The message was from the mother of a fifteen-year-old boy named Kevin.

Her message to me was a request for an immediate appointment for her son who had just been released from a Methodist hospital in Fort Worth. Stomach pains were causing him tremendous grief. She was concerned and confused when doctors could not diagnose her son's serious health problem. Kevin and his family had declined exploratory surgery.

Kevin sat on my table looking frail and bewildered and tried to stay calm and brave as he explained symptoms of cramping pains in his abdomen that grew from moderate to severe every time he ate food. He also told me that he had lost over fifteen pounds mainly because he was afraid to eat for fear the uncomfortable pain would interrupt him at school.

I felt sure that I would be able to eliminate the problem. I had a good suspicion what might have seized his immune system. The four of us were in my office when the boy and his parents suddenly began speaking at once. I could feel myself distancing from the pack as my mind traveled out to the small town where Kevin grew up. I knew that town well because my son was a student at the same school Kevin attended. I heard myself asking Kevin if he worked in the food business and knew immediately that the bacteria he had contracted was from the place where he worked.

I had to be tricky. I did not want his parents to freak out and leave the room, taking my client with them. My job was that of a healer. If I told the three of them about my sudden knowing, I might be called a charlatan rather than a healer of God. There was obviously a bacterial infection lurking somewhere within his body causing serious stomach problems. I asked Kevin if he would be willing to take nutrition in the form of pills. I explained that the pills were made from whole foods and told him they were neither addicting nor harmful in any way. I realized the dilemma with taking nutrition to solve a health problem was targeting the underlying issue before choosing which herb to take. In his case, because I knew he worked in the fast-food industry, I was pretty sure the bitter herbs and a strong probiotic would ease his growling stomach and nonstop pain.

Kevin was at a crossroads; he could go back to the hospital and have exploratory surgery or try something unconventional. I assured him that he would not need to continue taking the supplements once his body began to heal. I also assured him that he could beat this problem with patience, persistence, and nutritional supplements.

A mild to moderate enzyme that works fast is betaine hydrochloride, which also prevents bad breath, better known as halitosis, from undigested food in the body. I suggested he take this enzyme after meals to aid with digestion. I also suggested he began taking one choline daily to help clean out the bile ducts for delivery of enzymes to complete protein digestion. Betaine provides a good source of stomach acid for more rapid digestion of food. I know what you're thinking; I lean on supplementing with enzymes and choline. I admit it, I do, but it works and that is why I say take it.

Kevin was weak, and I knew he could use some iron. Iron can be difficult to digest in a pill form, but I knew he could advance from his sickness rapidly if he took iron for two to three weeks during this course of intense healing. I suggested he take two easy iron pills per week. I knew his heart wasn't into taking pills; my goodness, he couldn't even hold food down without feeling sick. Organic peanut butter and jelly will stick to the ribs. What kid doesn't enjoy that sandwich? Oatmeal or peanut butter will coat the stomach when it is necessary to take iron. This food will help you avoid feeling nauseous, as will eating bits of a scraped apple.

Foods high in protein take longer to digest. I suggested eliminating all red meat products until his digestive problems were better. Eliminating proteins, especially red meats, will help simplify the digestive system. Normal digestion of protein is a twenty-four-hour process. If digestion is delayed or some unexpected bacteria such as parasites burrow into the intestines, there can be a serious problem. This is precisely what had happened to Kevin.

My discovery for Kevin was not an unusual finding in the busy fast-food world we live in. He had contracted tapeworms. It is possible that the meat he had ingested had tapeworm larva in its muscles. This larva incubates in your intestines and can develop into adult tapeworms. Tapeworms must die before they are excreted from bowel movements, or they can hang out inside the intestines where they can live up to thirty years and grow to eighty feet long. Tapeworms attach themselves to the intestinal wall causing irritation and inflammation. Kevin told me he felt like there was a rock inside of his stomach. Parasites were invading his small intestine and causing gas pain and digestive problems. Adults and children who have similar problems can benefit from eating enzymes.

Depression, headaches, and stomachaches are all symptoms of a parasite infection. This was not a quick fix. He needed artemisia to dry out the parasites and L-cystine to kill off the eggs.

I could tell Kevin was a willing candidate for natural healing, and I truly had compassion for him and his mother, who appeared to be at her wits end over her son's deterioration in health and weight loss. I explained to him as thoroughly as possible that the human body is like a machine and will run smoothly if it is fed the correct fuel.

I asked this young man what he ate on a regular basis, and he began explaining to me that he worked at a local hamburger joint in the small town he lived in. He told me that he ate a cheeseburger every day with pickles, onions, and loads of ketchup. He went on to say that he was given a free milkshake with every meal he ordered. "Oh golly gee," I yelped. "Let's add a little glue to your meals to be sure that your stomach is entirely gummed up." I kept the description of parasites on the down low but remembered Dr. Versendaal's analogy of fast foods gumming up the automobile's gas tank. Kevin's eyes got as big as the hamburgers he ate when I told him my hypothesis. He got the point and had no choice but to follow my directions and get to feeling better fast.

I suspected there was more to the story than he cared to admit. I picked his brain until he finally remembered the beginning of his health crisis. He admitted to having diarrhea for weeks on end, which is a real warning flag. Intestinal problems and stomach pains are a serious symptom of intestinal amoebas. The reason laboratories don't always find parasites in a fecal stool sample is because the parasites are alive and not willing to budge. These unfortunate people who ate contaminated food have no idea how to stop IBS or constipation.

Though Kevin's father was hesitant to agree with my theory, he purchased the product for his son to give this treatment a go. Kevin continued the treatment for six cycles of the moon waxing and waning. He took a combination of bitter herbs far beyond the days he no longer felt the symptoms. Be assured: all parasite eggs must be eliminated before the problem is completely solved.

I sensed that Kevin was having some stress issues in keeping up with his grades, homework, trombone practice, and the part-time job he took at the fast-food restaurant. I told him to pick up a one-ounce bottle of liquid chamomile at the health-food store to calm his nerves. He dropped his head and started laughing as if he were amazed and relieved at the same time.

I insisted he packed his school lunch to include berries, almond butter, rice chips, and fresh vegetables. I instructed him to lay completely off of the fast food for at least one hundred and twenty days. He looked disappointed when I told him to put a halt on his beloved cheeseburgers. The patty may have had parasite eggs that were flash frozen in the factory and then delivered from the meat market to the restaurant. He grunted at my comment, but I knew he believed me. Young people are the best when it comes to getting well fast.

I can sense that when people are sick and tired of being sick and tired, they will search for answers when their backs are to the wall. I was happy to help, but the real work would be for Kevin to make dramatic changes in his eating habits.

I laid down the nutritional law that was mandatory for him to get well. He agreed to stop all junk food, including dairy, which was causing more mucus in his sinuses than he cared to admit. Kevin said he would do some serious food altering during his healing phase.

Six months after my first visit with Kevin, I received a letter from him telling me he had gained back the fifteen pounds that he had lost during his illness. It was so good to hear he was digesting and eliminating without pain. I was impressed with the progress he had made simply by altering his diet and taking healing supplements. His life was back on the fast track, and though I am sure he is eating an occasional cheeseburger, I bet he knows what to do if he ever bites into one that is not well cooked.

Praying It Forward

In the same way, the Spirit helps us in our weakness. We do not know what we ought to pray for, but the Spirit himself intercedes for us with groans that words cannot express.

— Romans 8:26 (NIV)

These words chosen in Praying It Forward were channeled from my spirit in a meditative state to bring forth healing for you. Feel free to alter them as only the Creator knows your needs. As long as you are coming from love and willing to receive, you are praying it forward.

Holy Creator, giver of health and life, thank you for the spirit's revelation at this perfect time in our lives. Thank you, conscientious farmers, who are working to save the planet; thank you for eliminating the chemicals from our food. Thank you for the harvesting and shelving of organically grown plants.

I bless my food at every meal by offering it pure white light before I eat it. I focus awareness on the importance of thinking pure thoughts, and I understand that thoughts have energy to help me digest my food.

Thank you, dear one, for offering me suggestions to help my digestive problems. May they be corrected now and always. Bless those less fortunate who are experiencing pain and indigestion. Bring healing to those who need help with digestion. They are healed, we are happy, and all are blessed.

Golden Rules

Stress and anxiety are choices that we make,
ways that we choose to process events.

— Dr. Wayne Dyer

Herbs and vitamins described in each chapter are not meant to replace any medicine prescribed by your medical doctor. Be sure to follow relevant directions on product labels and consult your pharmacist or physician before using herbs and natural supplements.

Symptoms of digestive issues can be incognito; headaches, insomnia, depression, irritability, and constipation are all symptoms of digestive issues.

According to Marilyn and Harvey Diamond, coauthors of the amazing, life-changing book *Fit for Life*, the human being's digestive system runs a silent clock that strikes an eating and digestive cycle from 12:00 p.m. to 8:00 p.m. It rolls a rhythm of absorption and use of food from 8:00 p.m. to 4:00 a.m. The body then kicks into elimination from 4:00 a.m. to 12:00 p.m. the following day. These cycles are responsible for our life force energy. Now you know that with a little help from your friends, enzymes, you can enhance all three cycles. Melatonin will help to adjust circadian rhythms and assist with sleep. Use sparingly and take in 2 to 5 mg only.

Go easy on your body by stopping all food consumption at 8:00 p.m. Take an enzyme before bedtime to help facilitate digestion, assimilation, and a good night's sleep.

Super Enzyme Caps and Wobenzym N are two popular and powerful enzymes. Begin using one or two with each meal, and if sleep is a problem, take one before bedtime.

Make one positive food change every week until you have trained your palate to enjoy a fresh salad or vegan sandwich for lunch. Do not wait until the last minute to choose your breakfast, lunch, or supper. Think healthy and think ahead. Begin combining digestible foods that produce enzymes for fast digestion. Carrots, parsley, couscous, and onions are a few foods to aid in digestion. Add splashes of lime with homemade salsa and use organically grown cilantro or vegetables when available.

Eat vegetables and rice as a combination for quick digestion to substitute a meat dish. Do not add carbohydrates in the form of rice or potatoes and bread with meat protein because it slows down digestion. If you slip up and a growling noise in your stomach persists accompanied by pain, take a teaspoon of arrowroot powder in water and a few drops of wormwood liquid.

Read labels and check condiments for high fructose corn syrup and artificial sweeteners. Candy and drinks that have colored dyes are merely there to catch your eye and slow the enzymatic process to a turtle's pace. High-sugar drinks decrease enzymes too and even worse cause hunger pains and acid stomach.

If you feel that you have eaten spoiled or contaminated food in any way, reach for the grapefruit seed extract and use ten to fifteen drops in warm water to destroy any bacteria or larva you may have eaten in your food. It is helpful to drink one tablespoon of apple cider vinegar in water if you experience diarrhea after eating a meal. Your body may be trying to purge some bacteria, so give it a helping hand.

If you have papaya fruit nearby, cut it and spoon out the black seeds. Eat one tablespoon of the papaya seeds after meals. These seeds hold precious enzymes and are strong enough to destroy any hidden amoeba eggs you may have contracted.

> Negative thoughts and stress sabotage our
> chances of excellent digestion.

> — Sherry Dell

Vision Blessing: The White Dove

> Let love and faithfulness never leave you; bind them around
> your neck, write them on the tablet of your heart.

> — Proverbs 3:3 (NIV)

Imagine you are sitting in a treetop. You are here to visit a gentle soul. Listen to the faint cooing of a dove. Breath ten long, deep breaths in and out until you feel connected to peace. White doves bring you feelings of peacefulness that stay with you the day long. This bird has joined you here on the tree branch to assure you that you are digesting properly. Enzymes are entering your bloodstream and flowing naturally into your stomach for safe and effective assistance with digestion.

The bird of peace is there for you each time you sit down to eat. The bird of peace is a reliable tool to remind you that trusting in the Spirit will help you relax and be confident that you are digesting the food you eat. Trust and know that you are digesting today. Say goodbye to the white dove and tell her you will come visit again soon.

Dove

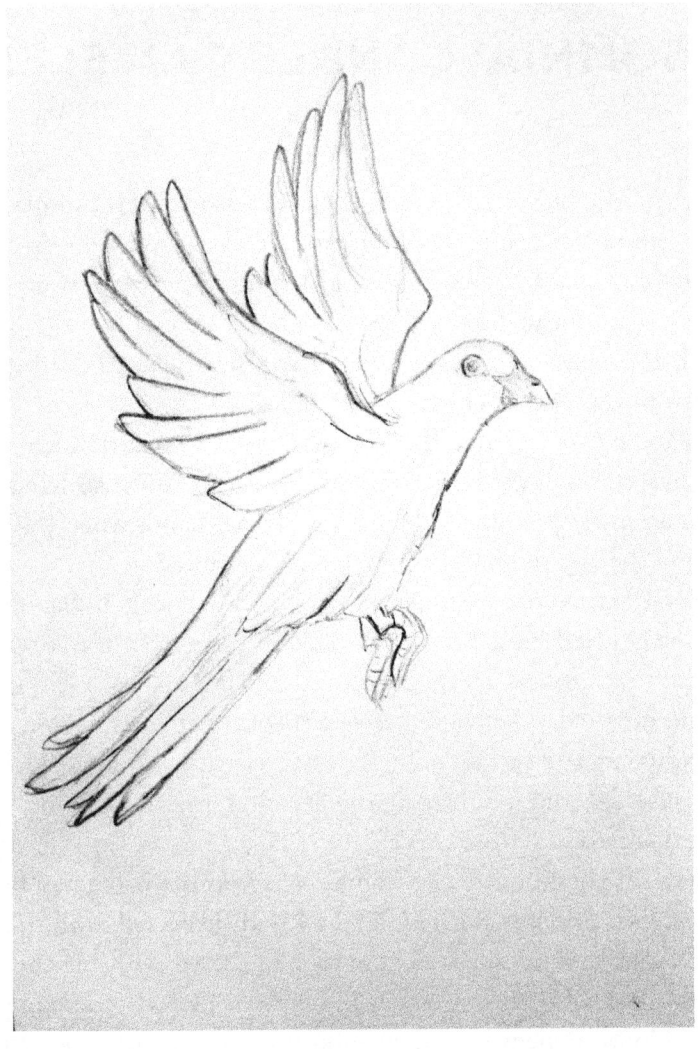

INSOMNIA: CANDLE CAN SLEEP

Many people think stress is the main reason for insomnia, but stress can be a side effect of indigestion and constipation. Anxious thoughts can slow down digestion, leaving a person too upset to maintain an optimal pH balance. Acidic blood can fray the pineal gland, the majesty of sleep. Once the pineal gland is disturbed, peaceful sleep doesn't come easy!

Candle came to my office looking like a wet cat that had been prowling through the back streets of New York. She was lying face down on my table with her blond head in her hands when I walked into my therapy room to begin our first consultation.

Candle was covered in perspiration and had tears in her eyes as she slowly lifted herself from the table to offer me a blank stare. I put my arms around her shoulders and told her to keep a stiff upper lip and hold back the tears. I have a theory that tears will relax an individual up to a certain point, but when crying is prolonged, tears can cause dehydration, leaving the person doing the sobbing weak and exhausted.

My first question to the woman was how often she had bowel movements. She was not regular, as I had suspected, and she did not eat meals when she was hungry. She shared with me that she had not had a bowel movement in fourteen days. I ordered up an old-fashioned remedy of two tablespoon of Epsom salt in one cup of warm water. The blond bombshell looked at me while shaking her head. "Have you lost your mind?" she asked.

"No, I have not." I replied, smiling. "You cannot go on acting so irresponsibly. Your appendix may rupture."

She implied that she did not think she was being irresponsible, but I informed her that we all must have an obligation to our health.

After two weeks of continuous constipation, it was time to do something serious to open the floodgates. "Why haven't you added fiber to your diet?" I asked. She responded that she hadn't wanted to gain weight. I explained to her that nothing speeds weight loss quicker than having regular bowel movements. I began to sense insecurity and a lack of confidence. Candle stood up and looked into my office mirror. She began to comb her hair and pucker her lips. I wondered why a pretty lady like this seemed so insecure and anxious. I could relate to her in many ways.

I saw that she was a pleaser, and I looked at her hand and saw a tattoo that read "Mom." It wasn't just a guess that had me on the edge of my seat. I had to know if she had lost her mother when she was a small child. When I asked her, she looked away and said, "My mother gave me up for adoption when I was three years old." "Love yourself and forgive her," I said. I could only hope she knew what I meant by saying these words. I asked her what she did to keep her weight down, and she responded with words that truly hurt my ears. Chemical sweeteners are in no way going to come near any of my client's mouths—not today, not ever. I defend their health and bend the rules as much as possible, but this was breaking the nutritional law.

The use of chemical sweeteners causes bloating and swelling, lowers the immune system, and weakens the kidneys. As a matter of fact, I have notice swelling in and around the eyes, mouth, and stomach for clients who get sidetracked and use this product as a weight-loss aid. When she asked me about fiber foods, I told her my favorite was a bowl of granola that consisted of one-half teaspoon of wheat germ, sunflower seeds, some lecithin granules, bran and ground flax meal. I suggested sweetening the cereal with a touch of coconut sugar followed by a nice cup of ice-cold, unsweetened rice milk. I prompted Candle to take a few fenugreek capsules with her morning breakfast to ease inflammation in the colon. Fenugreek is also a great pill to keep your body believing it is plenty full. It aids in weight loss, and it is good to know that with this herb, yoga, and garcinia cambogia, anyone can keep the waistline trim and fit. Candle began to add fiber into her diet and eventually her irregularity disappeared.

Within three months her skin returned to a healthy glow because she stopped the chemical sweeteners. I had forgotten that she had restless leg syndrome (RLS) until she told that once she stopped the chemical drinks, her legs settled down. She sat up big and tall on my table and begged me for a sleeping remedy that would allow her eight hours of sleep. She told me she had tried sleeping pills and that they kept her so hung over the next day that she could not read her manuscripts. Folic acid and B_{12} are on top of my list to take for a good night's sleep.

In the back of my mind, I thought her problem might be a circadian rhythm imbalance mixing up her nights and days. My suspicions were confirmed when she explained to me that she kept irregular hours due to her erratic work schedule. I quickly wrote on her chart a protocol to rotate the supplements vitamin A (no more than 1,000 IU per day) and vitamin D (dry, not oil capsule). I believe that vitamin A and D should be used sparingly so that the body does not store them since they are both fat-soluble vitamins.

Melatonin will help to improve a condition known as seasonal affective disorder (SAD), a vitamin D deficiency from lack of sun. We must allow our magnificent bodies to have rest on a regular basis. The body must be trained to rest, and it must have time to rejuvenate before we crank it up to begin our daily or nightly routine.

Linus Pauling, Nobel Prize winner and author of *Vitamin C and the Common Cold*, suggests taking large amounts of vitamin C daily to purge allergies and toxins from the body. Taking large doses of vitamin C will help to accelerate and support liver function to charge our immune systems. I enjoy taking vitamin C with bioflavonoids to strengthen the capillaries in the eyes and ears. Spread the doses of vitamin C therapy out and don't forget to drink a glass of water with each pill.

Among other acupressure points, I tested Candle's digestion, which failed miserably. I asked if she was taking prescriptions for energy and sleep, and she admitted to taking muscle relaxers, pain pills, and sleeping pills due to her pressing schedule as an up-and-coming actress. I asked her if she starred in *Valley of the Dolls*, and she cracked up laughing. For those of you too young to remember, prescriptions pills were known as dolls in the late seventies.

Today the lovely Candle is not dependent on any dolls except vitamins and nutrition. I reminded her that occasional constipation could be remedied by drinking a hot cup of tea or coffee followed by a cup of ice-cold water to create peristalsis motion for activation of the colon.

Antioxidants in the organic form of pomegranates, parsley, and cilantro help remove metabolic waste products from the blood and interstitial fluids. Oxidative stress may damage cells and DNA causing heart disease, type 2 diabetes, and cancer. The metabolic organs are involved with circulating and cleansing our precious fluids. Antioxidant foods are colorful and come in a variety of fruits and vegetables. While organic grapes and berries are helpful with eliminating waste from the body, they also stir up an abundance of energy. Think about eating the color of the rainbow, and you will capture the full spectrum of antioxidant foods.

Candle has no more desire to take stimulants for energy. Instead, she keeps a bowl of berries and a glass of lemon water near her side whenever she is rehearsing on the set. Her skin has returned to a healthy glow, she stopped the chemical sweeteners, and she is happy and reunited with the person she once was before her lifestyle as a superstar and jet-setter became too difficult to manage. Candle is now loving herself and no longer burning herself at both ends.

Love yourself, let go of resistance, and your
spirit will make music with your soul.

— Sherry Dell

Praying It Forward

Be careful for nothing; but in every thing by
prayer and supplication with thanksgiving let
your requests be made known unto God.

— Philippians 4:6 (NIV)

These words chosen in Praying It Forward were channeled from
my spirit in a meditative state to bring forth healing for you. Feel
free to alter them as only the Creator knows your needs. As long as
you are coming from love and willing to receive, you are praying it
forward.

Should you be one of the many people who have trouble sleeping,
I have a feeling that you know what it means to pray it forward.

Dear God, creator of all good things and divine healer, thank
you for allowing me to sleep tonight. I bask in faith as I send unto
the heavens my request to fall asleep. I am confident I will drift into
a sound sleep. Thank you for a perfectly glorious day and a peaceful
night.

I am confident I am investing in the magic of sleep. I am thrilled
to know that good things come to me as I continue to heal with
food and thought. I am thinking more positively every day. I enjoy a
healthy routine and treat my body as a temple of God. I am blessed
with awesome sleep. I am healed. I am loved. I am all that I hope to be.

Thank you, angels, and thank you prayer givers and friends who
have joined the golden chain of healing. I am blessed to connect to
the infinite wisdom of calmness, serenity, and peace.

I relax in knowing that I can sleep. It is so. Sleep is my best
friend.

Golden Rules

Herbs and vitamins described in each chapter are not meant to replace any medicine prescribed by your healthcare provider. Be sure to follow relevant directions on product labels and consult your pharmacist or physician before using herbs and natural supplements.

I focused on isolated problems with the sleepy-eyed client. I asked her to stretch out her hamstrings by pressing against the wall with both hands and moving one foot backward as far as possible to bend into a lunge stretch for release of lactic acid in long thigh muscles. This stretch improves sleep, so do it before laying down to sleep. To relax muscles and feed the bones, I suggested she begin taking one teaspoon of bone meal powder mixed with an extra tablespoon of ground flaxseed meal. This remedy can be sprinkled onto applesauce or on a small bowl of oatmeal for a quick bite of health before bedtime. The calcium in the bone meal not only relaxes the muscles, it quiets the mind to begin sleep.

I recommend insomniacs like Candle begin taking three linum B_6 supplements each day. This supplement supports the muscles' elasticity and oils creaky joints. Linum is flaxseed and converts to essential fatty acids that influence hormone production and help maintain healthy skin and nerve tissue. I prefer this superalkaline omega-3 fatty acid because it works well for vegetarians and will ensure that your liver is not overworked from animal fats. If push comes to shove and you are still not sleeping, it is mandatory to stop drinking coffee. If I can do it, anyone can. Although I told myself that I was drinking only organic coffee, I was still having interrupted sleep due to the acid pH balance in my blood. Finally, I switched to green tea and Tazo tea in the morning and can now sleep like a baby.

My client had succumbed to propping herself up on a pillow to sleep to help keep sinus drainage from waking her up. Try spraying your mouth with aloe vera juice before you retire to bed. As my parents would say, "Let us go say hello to our best friend, sleep."

My famous client was sleeping better by taking marigold bark in the evenings.

Take a good look at an alkaline food chart and write on a piece of paper the food choices you can easily integrate into your daily food schedule. By changing your diet to alkaline foods, you will get a head start on sleeping a good six to eight hours.

If you are a hard-case insomniac, follow Candle's direction on nightcaps to include one or two digestive enzymes before sleep and drink a warm cup of chamomile tea before bed. If you have aches and pain while lying in bed, get up and mix one tablespoon of bone meal powder and one tablespoon of flax meal. If you're still not having luck with sleep, you can pick up a bottle of Hyland's Calms Forté at the health store to quickly induce sleep. Only use as directed and do not use it with sleeping pills. Do not get dependent on any natural supplement because you are training the body to work on its own. Think about routine when it comes to eating and sleeping.

Discontinue caffeinated drinks completely and do not indulge in chocolate after five o'clock in the evening. If you are a caffeine addict or chocoholic, do not drink or eat it four to five hours before you try to sleep. Mugwort tea before bed is excellent for inducing sleep. Marigold bark capsules offer you a variety to choose from, so if one supplement doesn't seem to help go for the next in line. Take command over your stress and make yourself get into bed before midnight.

Eat organic blueberries and other antioxidant foods during the day or when you need extra energy. Have a bowl of oat bran cereal and bananas at night to wind down in the evening and sleep. Carbohydrates help to induce sleep. Take two inositol tablets if you awaken in the middle of the night—it is a sure bet to help you resume sleep as it coats the myelin sheath of the nerves.

Take vitamin A and D in low doses and purchase it in dry form, not oil, if possible. If you are on a gluten-free diet and feel it is working for you, congratulations! Substitute any bread or cracker and cereal with a trusted gluten-free grain or rice cakes.

If you wake up during the night with a sudden fear or anxiety, you are most likely drinking something that has caffeine in it. Check labels on all drinks and be aware of what they are sweetened with. Check to see if teas have caffeine and remember that most green teas are caffeinated.

Some people have nightmares when using melatonin, so if this happens to you, discontinue use. The liver must be able to filter all medicines, including natural vitamins. If you are having bad dreams, this is a sign of a congested liver. You should get to the health-food store, invest in apple pectin, and do the liver cleanse before using melatonin.

> Meditate on good things, think of good
> thoughts, and have a good night's sleep.

— Sherry Dell

Vision Blessing: Horse and Buggy Ride

I would like you to imagine that you are sitting in a horse-drawn carriage. Look outside the carriage windows and notice there is slight misting snow falling atop the trees and onto the ground. The horses pulling the carriage do not detour from the path. The Clydesdales slowly trot in a rhythm that is sure to repeat itself.

You hear a steady, slow, deliberate trot that is lulling you into serene peacefulness. Covered in warm blankets, you have no worries or cares in the world. You are at peace as you breathe in and out ten long, deep breaths. As the sound of horses' hoofs drifts into the distance, the silence of a soft, misting snow soothes you to your destination ... sleep.

Horse and buggy

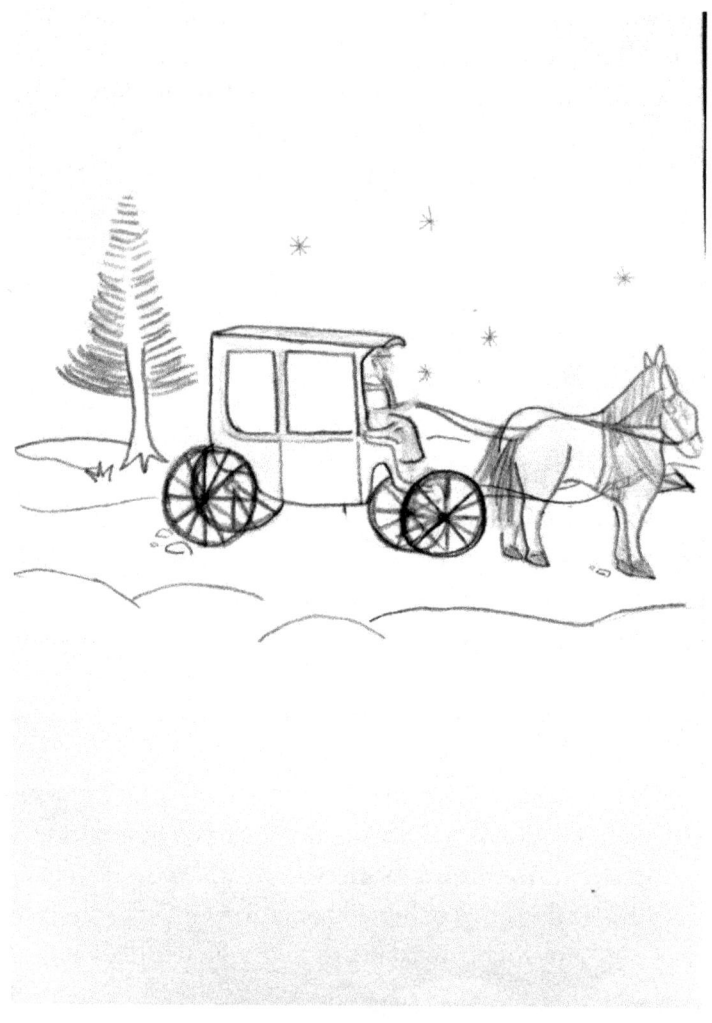

PANCREAS: THE DANCER SMILES

John walked into my office with a frown on his handsome face. He told me that he was bewildered by the incongruity between his blood work and the athlete he perceived himself to be. Red blood cells carry waste from the body via the kidneys and respiratory system. When the red blood cell number is low, it is a strong possibility the person is tired and anemic. More than fear of death, he had what I call F.O.C., or fear of change, and in most cases when illness is discovered, the change that a person fears more than anything in life is C.O.D, change of diet.

John's A1C numbers were shooting up to 6.4, and he told me that his primary physician was giving him ninety days to get the number down or start on insulin. I raised my hands up in the air as if to say, "Better late than never." I often wonder why it takes a catastrophic health crisis for a person to seek nutritional advice. In my opinion, it makes life easier to eat nutritious foods all along life's journey. It amazed me that this person was finally willing to investigate what he was doing wrong on his particular quest, and I applauded him for his courageous willingness to change. I pondered the idea that John was overwrought with toxins and might be unaware that certain foods he was accustomed to eating could be causing him big problems.

In my interview with him, I searched for his weakness in foods, and it didn't take ten minutes to discover that his favorite vice was drinking a half gallon of milk in the morning to start off his day. He then dined on cheeseburgers and salads at noon. He told me he had recently lost weight and finally admitted to feeling weak and run-down. When I heard this, I knew there was a possibility that he might be heading down the path of an immune disorder. I did not want to stack the deck for him, but many times elevated white blood cells will chase a trail of bacteria to a fire that is screaming to be extinguished. I asked him to name a few more of his favorite foods, and frankly, I was overwhelmed with his cheese chatter.

He said he frequently snacked on cheese nachos, ordered cheese on his sub sandwiches, ate cheese enchiladas, added cheese to his salads, and routinely served up a bowl of ice cream before going to bed at night. On weekends he would order cheese pizzas for his wife and friends when they hung out at his party barn on his ranch.

Without hesitation, I told him to cut out the C.R.A.P.—carbs, refined sugars, artificial foods, and processed meats.

This man loved horses and rode them almost every morning. On weekends, he jumped out of bed before sunrise to trail ride in the mountains, soaking up nature and wildlife. This country life was a city boy's dream come true. He had been blessed with an adventurous life surrounded by horses, goats, cats, and dogs, and he married his childhood crush when he was a teenager. His lovely wife, Karen, was kind and understanding and was willing to pay any price to help her talented husband survive.

I agreed with the dancer's wife and fan club; thousands of people dearly loved him and would miss him if he ever stopped performing. Now the dancer needed to know how to fuel his athletic body and control his blood sugar.

If the pancreas is too weak to support insulin production, the only sensible step to take is to clean the awesome four-pound liver using whole foods, herbs, and vitamins. The liver's home is above the pancreas and the small intestine, and the right kidney is below the pancreas.

I began my compelling theory by telling John that the next step to take was to change his diet. I hesitated to say the words but finally spoke earnestly and suggested elimination of all dairy products, even yogurt. In my opinion, the only chance he had to avoid a diabetic diagnosis was to chart out a diet change that consisted of steamed veggies, almond butter, rice, rice milk, organic fruits and vegetables, and plant-based protein. I suggested he purchase a centripetal juicer to begin juicing organic carrot, celery, and apple juice. I explained to him that adding phosphorus to his juice would aid in breaking down calcified dairy in his biliary system and pancreatic duct. Phosphorus makes up 1 percent of our body weight and is the second most abundant mineral in the body. It will aid in relieving middle back and shoulder pain when taken with organic apple pectin.

My advice to avoid dairy came to him as a complete shock, and I waited to continue speaking, hoping he would not resist the healing protocol that I so strongly recommended. I proceeded to outline a potential change of diet. I took a deep breath and told him straight to his honey brown eyes that before healing could begin, all animal protein must be eliminated from his diet. All meat had to be replaced with plant-based protein that is easier to digest, allowing rest and recuperation for all organs associated with digestion, especially the pancreas. I promised him that he could continue eating organic meat as soon as we accomplished our goals. I ordered up enzymes and covered almost every enzyme that came to mind. Lipase, amylase, bromelain, and pancreatic enzymes are supplemental enzymes that support liver, gallbladder, stomach, and pancreas activity. Food products are human-made foods such as Velveeta cheese, frozen dairy cones, powdered nondairy creamers, and thousands of tasty yet chemical-laden fake foods. When food products have been consumed by unsuspecting individuals like John, these digestive enzyme supplements can help with digestion and elimination of undigested food products. Acid forms in the stomach when food is not digested. If the pancreatic or bile duct have become hardened or blocked, there are no other saving supplements as awesome as choline and powdered inositol and the vegetable bitter melon.

We had no time to lose; we were on the medical doctor's watch list, and food and exercise were our valuable tools to use wisely. I told him some facts about recent studies on dairy. According to Dr. T. Colin Campbell, author of *The China Study*, casein found in dairy proved to be the most relevant cancer promoter ever discovered. Milk is 38 percent protein, and of that 38 percent, 80 percent is casein and 20 percent is whey. Casein is digested slowly, explained Dr. Campbell, son of a dairy farmer. His studies discovered growth of cancer cells could be turned on and off by regulating doses of casein.

He proved in many peer-reviewed studies that casomorphins, which are opioid peptides, are derived from the digestion of milk. Kevin nodded his head yes, indicating that he thoroughly understood that opioids were triggering his addictions to dairy. I went on to read another report aloud. The Yale Food Addiction Scale measures a person's dependence on cheese to be particularly high because it contains the addictive substance, casein. Casein, is present in all dairy and will trigger the brain's opioid receptors, which are linked to addiction. I used repetition to make my point and would not capitulate.

It is no wonder why unsuspecting humans become addicted to this sticky, tricky devilish delicacy (cheese) and the white wonder of America (milk). For the conclusion of the study, the doctor reported that whey in dairy is digested rapidly, causing a quick burst of insulin. Bursts of insulin stimulates IGF-1 (insulin growth factor) and has proven to promote cancer cell growth.

Astonished by this jarring information, John dropped his head as if he were ashamed and told me he was beginning to feel sick to his stomach. Then he laughed aloud at the paradox he had been living, believing he had escaped addictions by refusing to drink alcohol or take recreational drugs. He was determined to restore his health, and his concern grew as he remembered the words of his medical doctor, who had promised him insulin injections if his blood sugar did not lower within the next ninety days. I reminded him that kidney dialysis, an only option in many cases for diabetics whose kidneys can no longer function, was a dreadful exercise in life. He looked at me in a way that made me smile. John concurred; he could not continue eating in the manner to which he had become accustomed. Now he must kick a silent addiction of toxic foods.

I had to continue preaching from my soap box because I know human nature. Some people will do well for a week or so and then fall back into old eating habits that got them into trouble in the first place. I told him the story about the man who had an aching stomach until he drank a quart of milk. When his stomach started hurting again, or when the milk became soured in his stomach, he had to drink it over and over to put out the fire.

It is almost impossible to eliminate dairy from the diet without taking a form of enzymes to help digest the sludge of bacteria. The real trick is to coat the stomach with slippery elm or okra pepsin before going to sleep at night. I suggested he begin to take the papaya enzymes, and when I handed him the bottle, he popped two in his mouth to chew as we continued our conversation. I was looking for more clues to solve the answers as to why this athlete's blood sugar was skyrocketing.

He finally admitted that when he needed extra energy, he hit the vending machines during, before, and after his dance rehearsals. He attributed this habit to his childhood. He would grab a few bars of candy when he left school to walk directly to the studio where he studied ballet and jazz dance. Like a kid in a candy store, his adult child kept the memory alive, and he was convinced he could not live without satisfying his sweet tooth. My job was to convince him he could not live by continuing to subsist on his current diet. We both agreed that eating to live was the best option to take.

John had to get started on a liver cleanse as soon as possible. I suggested that since he was in a bit of a hurry to detox, he should begin drinking dandelion tea in the range of three to four cups per day. He told me that was no hill for a stepper. I held back a belly laugh and promised him that he could use stevia organic sweetener by the company SweetLeaf.

John's lips began to form a Cheshire cat grin as he rocked back in his chair and told me he believed he could make this change happen. I told him that all milk solids had to be eliminated, including milk chocolate. He grabbed at his chest like I had shot him in the heart with a poison arrow. This man was a lovely person, and I knew he had the zest for life that was required to complete the C.O.D. With my fingers crossed, I hoped his Irish luck would continue to manifest years to his life and joyful entertainment to ours.

Praying It Forward

I have set the LORD always before me. Because
He is at my right hand, I shall not be moved.

— Psalm 16:8 (NIV)

These words chosen in Praying It Forward were channeled from my spirit in a meditative state to bring forth healing for you. Feel free to alter them as only the Creator knows your needs. As long as you are coming from love and willing to receive, you are praying it forward.

There is nothing more devastating than news of debilitating health for yourself, loved ones, or friends. In the likeness of a perfect image of everlasting life, there is spirit lodging in a physical body. The spirit has a will to continue life and has been known to make its presence known even after death. My prayer for those who are struggling with a change of diet is for them to meditate on the sweetness of life. I appreciate the kind acts of others and admire the strength and discipline I have acquired.

I am thankful for the strength and willpower for those of us who have controlled our blood sugar. I appreciate the joy healing brings to us minute by minute, day by day, and year by year. I thank God, heaven, earth, pine trees, wildlife, and blue skies. Thank you, Creator, for allowing us to live life as sweetly as possible every day. Thank you for helping us care and pray for others who haven't the courage to change their diets. Thank you for clean bodies where our spirits can reside. May God bless and protect small children who are born diabetic. We thank you for healing children. We give our gratitude for complete healing and appreciate the excellent quality of life we receive each and every day.

Thank you for giving us the strength to understand our condition and the willpower to improve it. Bless those who have a difficult time resisting sweets and fried foods. Give hope to all of us who have the same challenges as John and bless our food from morning to night.

Thank you, readers, for making better food choices and remembering John, who loved life and did his best to overcome high blood sugar.

Golden Rules

If slaughterhouses had glass walls, everyone would be a vegetarian.

— Sir Paul McCartney

Herbs and vitamins described in each chapter are not meant to replace any medicine prescribed by your healthcare provider. Be sure to follow relevant directions on product labels and consult your pharmacist or physician before using herbs and natural supplements.

Put your Elton John hat on and throw Janis Joplin feathers around your neck. Celebrate, and think of the vegan life as saving you tons of problems down the long and winding road of pancreatic illness.

Some of the symptoms associated with pancreatic problems include: feelings of indigestion; cramping after meals; large amounts of gas; foul-smelling gas or stools; floating or greasy, fatty stools; experiencing pain in right or left shoulder and middle-to-low back; and craving sweets and carbohydrates after eating a large meal.

The pancreas is like an orchid—it is rare and very delicate and needs tender loving care in order to continue around-the-clock digestion. Nurture this flower and understand that this organ needs to run a marathon for you every day. Eating refined sugar does nothing but shock and jolt this beauty into wilting. If the bile duct has been clogged with hardened bile, the pancreas demands to be fed carbohydrates and sugars.

The suggested change of diet almost always works. Once this sweet organ blossoms into full bloom, the fragrance is long-term health. Read all packages for sugar and don't allow any to enter your mouth; substitute dairy with soy-free, non-GMO products; and do not eat animal protein for twelve consecutive months to give your pancreas a break. Indulge in plant protein, eat small meals, and think delicious thoughts daily.

This dairy-worshiping nation has catapulted over the top of the food pyramid, believing that cow's milk is a necessity for supporting health. It is almost impossible to eliminate dairy from your diet without taking enzymes on a daily basis. Wobenzymes N is a strong enzyme, so play it safe and begin to introduce the amount you take into your body slowly. If you are experiencing a sensitive or painful stomach when lying down or after eating a big meal, this tells me that you could be halfway into the ulcer zone, if not there already. Should this be the case, you may heal an ulcerated stomach by taking okra pepsin at night on an empty stomach, last thing before you go to bed. Chew pepsin enzymes and slippery elm during the day to rebuild a thin stomach lining.

Bromelain enzymes may also help to eliminate toxic sludge and soak up stomach acid. Papaya enzymes are one of the first natural edible enzymes that graced the shelves of health-food stores in the early seventies. If you have hypertension or take beta-blockers, then using papaya enzyme supplementation is not suggested due to its high potassium content.

The common bile duct and pancreatic duct work together inside the pancreas and empty enzymes into the small intestine so that the two can deliver insulin and bile for digestion of food. The small intestine cannot complete the job for digestion of protein if the pancreas is overloaded and unable to secrete enough enzymes for digestion of protein. These two organs work together for the digestion of fats, oils, protein, and simple or complex sugars. When the gallbladder is dry, the bile duct is limited in bile production; therefore, the pancreas will overcompensate and beg for sugar fixes all day long.

There is irony in cleaning this sweet organ with the use of cayenne pepper and bitter melon, two not-so-sweet herbs. Stay true to the vitamin choline and use powdered inositol or chewy inositol pills ordered from Standard Process. Take bitter melon in capsules to clean the pancreas and prevent parasites from living in the intestines. Beta carotene is also recommended as a healing vitamin, but do not take large doses.

Stop eating fried food and do grilled vegetables spiced with all-natural herbs like spike or lemon pepper. Substitute all fast foods with homemade salads or cabbage soups with rice and beans. Eat only organic fruits but eliminate apples and bananas because of their high sugar content. Eat seed- and grain-pressed bread with vegan butter. Add pineapples to chia seeds soaked in almond milk overnight to make a frozen smoothie. When dining with friends and guests, keep a mental focus of your longevity with a jack-o'-lantern grin like Kevin's. If you train your mind to be free of food addictions, you can do a C.O.D. with joy and determination.

Remember to take a container of your favorite enzymes and vitamins with you so you can take them with each meal. Be it a café, a carnival, or a five-star restaurant, supplements are mandatory for healing.

Vision Blessing: Contented Swing

If hundreds, thousands, or even millions of human beings
embrace a new consciousness based on possibility; align their
actions with their intentions; and live by greater universal
laws of love, kindness, and compassion, a new consciousness
will emerge—and we'll experience true oneness.

— Dr. Joe Dispenza, *You Are the Placebo*

Follow me with your imagination down a cobblestone path
that leads to a road. Stop directly in front of a sign fastened above a
tree that reads "Your Health" and points toward a path you happily
follow. This path expands into a broader street that is paved and
bordered with yellow tulips. As you continue walking, visualize a
wooden swing looped around a large oak tree fastened with two
strong ropes holding it in place. Walk over to the swing and sit
down on it. Take ten deep breaths as you pick up your feet and
kick off the ground with a slight swinging motion. You are happy,
and you have good reason to be. As you swing back and forth in a
steady motion, take notice just how relaxed and contented you have
become with the foods you have chosen to eat to improve to your
health. You are aware of all the precious gifts life has to offer you. As
you swing back and forth, realize that you have become less and less
attached to addictive foods that once controlled your life. Continue
swinging until you are sure that you have accepted this new diet
with confidence.

Swing attached to tree limb

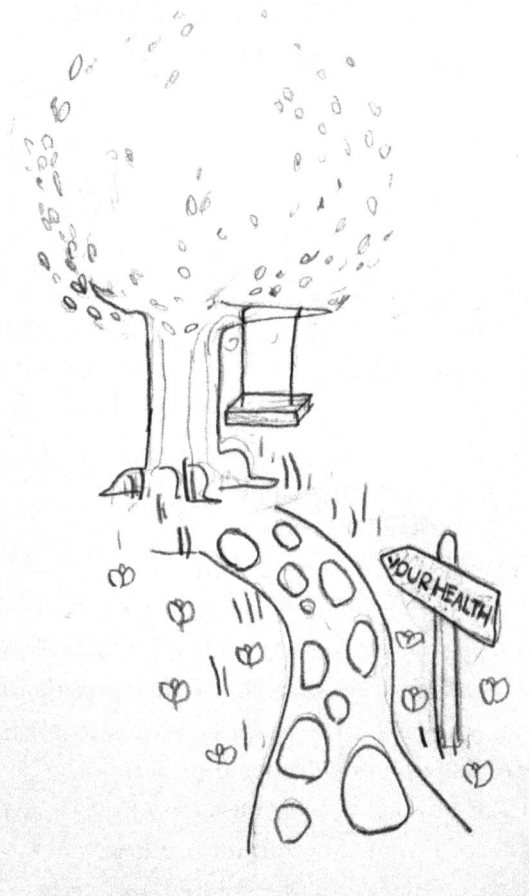

QUICK REFERENCE
TO SYMPTOMS

Chewing ice: People have the urge to chew ice when they are low on blood volume or lacking iron. Begin taking a parasite remedy and use one tablespoon of molasses twice a day to enrich blood. You may also search for a mild iron supplement that will not constipate you.

Knee pain: Unless injured, the knees swell with fluid if the kidneys are full of stones. Another cause of kidney stones can be calcium deposit in and around the cartilage. Take ten drops of Phosfood Liquid, drink organic apple juice, and use the vitamin Calsol distributed by Standard Process.

Butterfly nose: The nose will form a brown or discolored butterfly shape on the end of it when the spleen is not repairing blood cells. Use iron supplements, eat blackstrap molasses, and begin a parasite remedy as soon as possible. When the butterfly pattern has disappeared, you will know that the spleen is back to normal. If you have had cancer, take iron only in the form of foods.

Hip pain: The hips are the generators to a healthy heart. As we walk, the hips keep constant rhythm for our hearts to beat strong. When people have hip problems, they should stop dairy of any kind and take vitamin D. Use Phosfood Liquid and Collagen C for tissue repair. A kidney flush is a necessity. Discontinue drinking teas and sodas and drink alkaline water only for the best results. Slow down on magnesium if you are taking it daily.

Hernia in groin: Hernias are caused by excessive consumption of dairy. Kidney stones are very acidic and leave traces of acid in and around the hip and leg areas. Use kidney stone flushes after the hernia is repaired and do not drink sodas or use dairy products in excess.

Kidney stones: If you are having repeated kidney stones, hydrangea capsules, marshmallow root, ginger and uva-ursi are awesome herbs to help break down emulsified stones. Buy asparagus powder. Take one fourth package each night before bed. Asparagus powder is highly concentrated and will detox a person with toxic stones quickly. Drowsiness may occur after drinking it. Do not take more than one fourth package per day. It may take two to three weeks to break down these calcified, toxic stones, but like Mick said, "Time is on your side, yes, it is." After three weeks of taking the asparagus, follow up with a kidney stone flush.

GALLBLADDER FLUSH

Supplies for Flush

Organic apple juice: 2 gallons

Phosfood Liquid: 30 drops to 1 quart apple juice

Unisom (doxylamine succinate) or Hyland's Calms Forté

Epsom salt

Organic extra virgin olive oil

Organic lemons

Choline: 1 per day for two weeks before flush and two months following flush to ensure bile ducts remain open for completion of excess stones.

Add 30 drops Phosfood Liquid to 1 quart of organic apple juice and drink the 1-quart mixture for six days in a row. On day six, skip dinner and drink 2 tablespoons of Epsom salt dissolved into 1 cup water at 6:00 p.m. You must have bowel movement to clear the way for the passing of the stones.

Repeat the same Epsom salt mixture and drink again at 8:00 p.m.

It is permissible to flush any time during the day as long as you have not had any food three hours before you take the first Epsom salt drink.

You must have a bowel movement before continuing the flush.

At 10:00 p.m., make a cocktail of 8 ounces of olive oil and 4 ounces of freshly squeezed lemon juice, pour into a tightly sealed container, and shake vigorously. If you are not sure you can drink this cocktail all at once, divide the mixture into four doses. Drink one dose of the olive oil/lemon juice cocktail every ten minutes until you have consumed all four doses. Be sure to shake each dose well before drinking it. You may sip a bit of Sprite after the oil mixture if you are feeling an upset stomach. Less is best on Sprite—do not drink more than 2 to 3 ounces.

Go to bed and sleep on your right side with your knees pulled up to your chest if possible. If you are having trouble sleeping, take one Unisom or one Calms Forté to sleep soundly throughout the night.

Early the next morning, you should pass green and yellow gallstones as large as your thumbnail and as small as a pea. You will not feel any pain and will be amazed at the results. A natural diarrhea, not painful, will occur. If bowel movement is delayed, you must mix 1 or 2 tablespoons of Epsom salt in 2 ounces of warm water and drink again in the morning. Thousands of people have resolved their kidney stones with this method and avoided surgery.

LIVER FLUSH

The liver flush is exactly like the gallbladder flush except for the juice of a lemon is to be replaced with the juice of grapefruit juice. Read directions on gallbladder and substitute the juices as directed.

Note to those being treated with statins and high blood pressure medicine: Grapefruit is a contraindication to statins and should not be consumed. If, however, statins side effects are causing cramping in lower legs and loss of short-term memory, consult with your physician about using red yeast rice or CholestOff by Nature Made.

Be aware that one specific symptom of a sluggish liver is a trail of pain in the middle of the back or a sharp pinching twinge in the right or left side of the neck and shoulders. Apple pectin is a calorie-free substitute for apple juice used in liver and gallbladder cleanses. Take one a day to keep the doctor away.

KIDNEY FLUSH

Prepare for a kidney flush by using one Chi Asparagus Pack per night for two or three weeks. Kidney stones are solid masses of crystals that contain undigested calcium. Use small amounts of powdered magnesium, but do not overdo this mineral as it will rob calcium and precious fluids from your body. This is a good time to introduce the mineral phosphorus into your diet. Use six to ten drops in water or apple juice each day to soften stones and increase urination.

Ingredients needed are: powdered magnesium, liquid asparagus packs, choline, and 2 cans or ½ pound of asparagus.

Drink 8 ounces of apple juice per day or take 2 apple pectin pills for seven days. Add 1 choline to your vitamin protocol daily. Use small amounts of powdered magnesium (no more than ¼ teaspoon) mixed in distilled water and add no more than 20 drops of Phosfood Liquid to juice or water. *It is extremely important to discontinue all dairy.*

On the sixth day of the cleanse, skip dinner and sauté one pound of asparagus to eat or open two cans of asparagus. After eating the asparagus, drink six 12-ounce original Coca Colas. Be sure to read the ingredients on the Coke bottle—it should contain sugar as an ingredient, not high fructose corn syrup.

Note to diabetics: Don't forget you can still do this flush by using S.Pellegrino water in place of the Cokes. I would love to encourage diabetics to stop using artificial and aspartame sweeteners.

MASTER CLEANSE

Mix together in 1 gallon of distilled water the juice of 4 organic lemons, a pinch of cayenne pepper, and 6 tablespoons grade B maple syrup. Drink this water for one week and try to limit your food intake. Many of my clients simply fast on the sweet-and-sour water only. Use this master cleanse to detoxify your body and lose weight.

REMEDIES FROM THE KITCHEN

Eat licorice or drink the tea; it has a calming effect and is an aphrodisiac to both men and women. Licorice also stimulates adrenals. Do not drink the tea at night unless you plan on staying up late.

Take withania liquid, 6 to 7 drops in warm lemon and honey water. Withania is an Ayurveda herb that calms the mind and stills a nervous condition.

Use small doses of powdered magnesium in warm water. Some brands will provide calcium with magnesium. Use in small doses and never take an abundance of calcium. If you are over forty years old and experience a worsening of joint pain, discontinue calcium/magnesium for a week and then resume use in smaller proportions. Magnesium hydrates the colon using our precious interstitial fluids. It's worth mentioning that while magnesium is an excellent mineral to relax the muscles and purge lactic acid, too much of this wonder vitamin can dry out ligaments and cause dependency for bowel movements.

Too much calcium can be stored on the outside of the bones. If you are taking calcium to relax and your hands or fingers have knots on them, it is possible that you are not digesting nor assimilating the calcium supplement that you are using. Try using the herb oat straw as a calcium supplement. Remember that a little goes a long way.

Drink chamomile tea and take chamomile capsules to relax the mind. Take Saint John's wort for depression and valerian to induce sleep.

Avoid foods that have preservatives in them, such as prepared frozen dinners with MSG. MSG can cause anxiety and reduces feel-good hormones. Cook homemade dishes and freeze them for easy meals when in a hurry.

Korean ginseng is an excellent elixir and mood lifter. It is also a good supply of quick energy. It tones heart muscles much like hawthorn, and it is a mild aphrodisiac for men and women.

Use lavender to calm the nerves. Shake a few drops on a scarf or handkerchief and tie around your neck to sniff a delightful fragrance of enhanced serenity throughout the day.

Drink gotu kola tea for mental clarity. If you take it in pill form, begin with one in the morning. This product is very strong and will relax you too much if you do not begin the treatment slowly.

In the Cupboard for the Kidneys

If the kidneys have debilitated into Bright's disease, also called acute or chronic nephritis, eat nothing but watermelon for at least five days. Take five days off, eat your normal diet, and repeat the watermelon cleanse again for another round of five days.

Kidney problems can improve by eating red bell peppers and asparagus and drinking parsley tea.

Mix together 2 cups of red grape juice and ½ teaspoon of cream of tartar. Drink and urinate old toxins from the bladder and kidneys.

Boil ½ cup watermelon seed in 1 quart distilled water, add ¼ teaspoon of magnesium/calcium powder strain, and drink 1 cup daily.

Take juniper berry capsules three times daily to purge kidneys and keep the heart strong. Drink blue vervain tea to reduce static in ears and improve hearing.

In the Cupboard for Pinworm Infections

For children under twelve years of age:
Eat 1 sour pickle per day and drink cucumber juice or eat the cucumber with a thin layer of mustard spread over crackers.

Eat 6 to 7 saltine crackers chased with pickle juice; drink 2 ounces per day.

Grind 24 pumpkin seeds with a pumice stone and make a paste with almond butter and honey. Spread the paste over rice crackers and eat this treat daily. Pumpkin seeds will eliminate the mother pinworms that live in the lower colon and burst open when laying her eggs. Research tells us the mother pinworm can lay over one thousand eggs at a time. This parasite is inhaled through the nose just like pollen. It triggers a similar allergic response, making one's nose itch. If untreated, this parasite can cross the intestinal wall, enter the bloodstream, and soak up precious fluids.

Like allergies, pinworms can bring the immune system down causing tiredness, irritability, and hyperactivity. Add these symptoms up and you get a lack of concentration in children and a big fancy emotional label know as ADHD. Add 6 drops of lavender oil in the bath and apply Thieves or Purification Oil in small amounts on the child's belly.

Eat raisins for building blood and prunes for proper elimination. Disguise the raisins and prunes in a cupcake mixture. Be clever—most children resist treatment at first, so do not even explain to them why they need the treatment! The best medicine for children is bed rest and red blood builders. Animal Parade with iron is great for stilling the mind and increasing memory. Focus Factor is a great supplement for a hyper child. Try using blackstrap molasses for building red blood. Red beans are also healing for anemia.

Eat figs or buy fig powder and mix with applesauce and eat 2 tablespoons each night before bed. Standard Process sells Zymex II, which is pure fig powder.

Try to keep the child's tiny hands away from candy and sweets and your big hand from handing it over to them. Substitute candy with clean, red, seedless grapes; strawberries; blueberries; dates; and figs. Pinworms are extremely activated when sugar enters the bloodstream.

Symptoms of a pinworm infection in children are picking at bottom of pants, picking nose, runny nose, ear infections, constipation, poop that looks like round golf balls, and teeth grinding while they sleep. Remember that pinworms thrive on the children's rich blood and fluids. The infection can make a child hyperactive, causing lack of concentration and learning disabilities. This infection can cause insomnia and cause adults to be irritable too.

Stay away from red dye drink, Coca Cola, snow cones, and powdered doughnuts. Dyes and chemicals in candies, cakes, and drinks only add fuel to the fire.

Purification Oil, distributed by Young Living, can be dabbed into the belly button of the infected child each night before sleeping. This oil is a topical solution only and can't be used internally. Do not miss a night, especially during the new and full moons.

In the Cupboard for Digestion

Green bell peppers help bring pepsin into the stomach to aid digestion.

Sage tea heated with basil and celery aid in protein digestion.

Ginger tea will soothe upset stomachs and aid with digestion.

Boil 1 tablespoon of alfalfa seeds per 2 cups water and steep for five minutes before drinking. This alkaline drink soaks up acid in the gut.

Arrowroot is especially good for upset stomach in the elderly or for a person who is extremely deficient in digestive enzymes due to a sick liver. Mix 1 tablespoon arrowroot with 3 tablespoons milk to make a paste. Then add the paste to water, stir well, and boil. Lemon juice or lime juice can be added for taste.

Applesauce or apple concentrate is especially good to improve digestion in children. Add sauce to fig powder for a nighttime snack.

Boiled zucchini is a magical vegetable for digestion. Wash and cut zucchini into small pieces, boil in clean water, and eat as a solo dish. Or toss in avocado oil, salt, and pepper and bake on a cookie sheet.

Take 1 tablespoon of vinegar in 1 cup of water to improve digestion and elimination of bacteria in the stomach and colon.

Drink the juice of 1 lemon daily in water to enhance your digestive system.

ALKALIZE AT HOME

For five days, beginning on day one of each month, mix together ¼ teaspoon baking soda to 1 cup water and the juice of half a lemon. Drink this alkalizing mixture in the morning on an empty stomach. Indulge in the morning the first five days of each month. This formula will alkalize the body, thereby keeping parasites from the colon and bloodstream. Alkalizing the blood also reduces the affinity for illness since bacteria thrives more readily in an acidic environment. Bacteria will not thrive in an alkaline environment as easily as it thrives in an acidic environment.

pH-Adjusting Foods

Acid-Forming Foods: chicken, dairy products, eggs, fish, grains, ham, lamb, pork (all forms), most nuts and seeds, and meat (beef, turkey, veal, and all store-bought processed foods).

Alkaline-Forming Foods: almonds, apricots, avocados, coconuts, figs, grapes, honey, lemons, maple syrup, molasses, raisins, Umeboshi plums, vegetables, all melons, and yogurt (soured products).

How to alkalize the liver by reducing heavy metals:

1 garlic clove
½ cup of almonds, walnuts, or sunflower seeds
1 cup packed cilantro leaves

2 tablespoons lemon juice
6 tablespoons olive oil

Optional: 1 jalapeno pepper for some zip

Add cleaned cilantro and olive oil in a blender and process until the cilantro is chopped. Add the rest of the ingredients and process to a lumpy paste. (You may need to add a touch of hot water and scrape the sides of the blender.) You can change the consistency by altering the amount of olive oil and lemon juice but keep the 3:1 ratio of oil to juice. (It freezes well, so you can make several batches at once.) You may also add nuts and spices to taste. Freeze the mixture in ice cube trays and eat one cube a day for three weeks.

CPSIA information can be obtained
at www.ICGtesting.com
Printed in the USA
BVHW081035170619
551190BV00007B/83/P

9 781982 227296